Misc...

THE

Second

BY

GILLIAN C. L. LACHELIN

*Reader and Consultant in Obstetrics and Gynaecology
University College London Medical School and
University College London Hospitals Trust*

Oxford   New York   Toronto
OXFORD UNIVERSITY PRESS
1996

Oxford University Press, Walton Street, Oxford OX2 6DP

Oxford   New York
Athens   Auckland   Bangkok   Bombay
Calcutta   Cape Town   Dar es Salaam   Delhi
Florence   Hong Kong   Istanbul   Karachi
Kuala Lumpur   Madras   Madrid   Melbourne
Mexico City   Nairobi   Paris   Singapore
Taipei   Tokyo   Toronto
and associated companies in
Berlin   Ibadan

Oxford is a trade mark of Oxford University Press

Published in the United States
by Oxford University Press Inc., New York

First edition published 1985
© Gillian C. L. Lachelin 1985, 1996

A catalogue record for this book is available from the British Library

Library of Congress Cataloging in Publication Data
(Data available)

ISBN 0 19 262613 2

Typeset by Palimpsest Book Production Limited,
Polmont, Stirlingshire
Printed in Great Britain on acid-free paper by
Biddles Ltd, Guildford and King's Lynn

Preface to the second edition

I am very grateful to many patients and friends who have made encouraging and helpful suggestions about the book, which I have incorporated into the new edition. I am particularly indebted to those who have written accounts of their miscarriages, which have, not unexpectedly, remained very vivid to them. I have included several of these personal accounts in the new edition as they illustrate very clearly many of the emotions that are felt by those unfortunate enough to experience one or more miscarriages.

London   G.C.L.L.
September 1995

Preface to the first edition

Miscarriages are unfortunately very common and very distressing. About one quarter of all women who become pregnant will have one or more miscarriages. A miscarriage is usually a devastating experience for the expectant parents, who are likely to experience a number of emotions including profound disappointment, fear of the process of miscarriage and about the future, sadness, self-pity, anger, grief, guilt, feelings of inadequacy, failure, and helplessness, and sometimes prolonged depression.

It is natural to seek an explanation for a miscarriage, and to wonder whether it was caused by a particular action. In fact, in most cases, the pregnancy could not have continued because of serious faults which occurred very early in development. Every one of us started life as a single cell, formed by fusion of a cell from each of our parents, and our bodies are eventually made up of millions and millions of highly specialized cells formed by repeated division from the first cell. A very small fault in cell division at an early stage can lead to failure in the normal development of the embryo or placenta and hence to a miscarriage. Given the complex and intricate mechanisms involved, it is amazing, when we think about it, that so many pregnancies come through this process at all. Likewise, it is not so surprising that so many pregnancies end in miscarriage.

In a few cases of miscarriage a cause can be found, but in most instances the specific cause will never be known. Once the initial grief has lessened, the parents may derive comfort from the fact that conception was possible in their case as the likelihood of a successful pregnancy is good even after two or more miscarriages.

The aims of this book are to try to give an understanding of the events of early pregnancy and of the factors that may adversely affect the development of the embryo, and to recognize and to explore the intense and prolonged distress that may result from a miscarriage. The causes, process, and effects of miscarriage are discussed, and advice is given about future pregnancies. It is hoped that, when a miscarriage does occur, the people involved will be able to cope better if they have some understanding of what is happening.

London G.C.L.L.
February 1985

Contents

1 *Introduction*
•••

Many people are unaware how frequently miscarriages occur and how much distress they may cause to the couples concerned. Probably between one in five or six, or more, of confirmed pregnancies end in miscarriage. This means that over 100 000 pregnancies end in miscarriages that are recognized as such in Britain each year, and that several hundred miscarriages occur each day. It is likely that the true rate of early pregnancy loss is in fact much higher than this—possibly more than three quarters of human conceptions are lost—but many of these losses occur before the women concerned are aware that they are pregnant, that is before a menstrual period is missed (see Chapter 6).

To the outsider a miscarriage may seem like a misfortune that the couple should soon get over but to the parents, the loss of a pregnancy, even at a very early stage, may be utterly devastating and the miscarriage may have profound and prolonged emotional effects on them (see Chapter 5). Greater understanding of the causes and processes by which miscarriages occur, and greater awareness of the parents' needs and feelings, may help to alleviate the couple's distress to some extent.

The terms 'miscarriage' and 'abortion' are used interchangeably by doctors and others to mean the loss of a pregnancy from the uterus (womb) in the early months of pregnancy. Many people find this upsetting as they feel that abortion implies deliberate termination of a pregnancy, but as the terms are used like this in practice they have been used in this way in this book, with appropriate adjectives where necessary to make the meaning clear (see below).

It is important to understand the terms that are used to describe the length of time that a woman has been pregnant. The terms 'weeks' gestation' and 'weeks of pregnancy' are used to mean the number of weeks since the first day of the woman's last menstrual period, assuming that she has a roughly 28 day menstrual cycle,

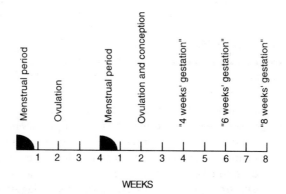

Figure 1 Diagrammatic representation of a menstrual cycle and a cycle in which conception has occurred.

as the actual date of conception is not usually known. Thus 15 weeks of pregnancy (or 15 weeks' gestation) means 13 weeks after conception, as ovulation and conception usually occur 2 weeks before the next period would have occurred, that is on about day 12–14 of a 28-day cycle (see Figure 1).

The definition of miscarriage used to be the loss of a pregnancy from the womb before 28 weeks' gestation. This is no longer appropriate as many babies born before 28 weeks of pregnancy now survive and develop normally. Babies born at 26 weeks' gestation have a better than one in two chance of survival in a modern neonatal intensive care unit. The term miscarriage is now usually used to mean loss of a pregnancy before 20–24 weeks' gestation.

The duration of pregnancy is divided descriptively into three trimesters or terms—the first trimester being up to 14 weeks, the second from 14 to 28, weeks and the third from 28 weeks until delivery. Miscarriages that occur before 14 weeks are known as first trimester miscarriages and those that occur after 14 weeks as second trimester miscarriages.

Threatened miscarriage/abortion means that the woman experiences vaginal bleeding during the early months of pregnancy, usually in the first trimester. The bleeding may be slight or heavy and may or may not be accompanied by lower abdominal discomfort and backache. It is a common problem and is discussed further in Chapter 3.

Spontaneous miscarriage/abortion indicates that the miscarriage occurred naturally and that it was not induced.

Complete miscarriage/abortion means that the fetus (developing baby), placenta (afterbirth), and amniotic sac (membranes)—have all been expelled from the uterus, and that the uterus is empty and a curettage (scrape) is not necessary. Very early miscarriages, before 7 weeks' gestation, are usually complete.

Incomplete miscarriage/abortion implies that only some of the placental tissue and membranes have been expelled from the uterus and that some tissue remains in the uterus. This means that there is a risk of further bleeding and of infection, and that curettage is required.

Missed abortion (or early embryonic demise—the preferred term in the United States) indicates that the fetus has died but that a miscarriage has not yet occurred. A missed abortion can often be diagnosed with an ultrasound scan.

Septic abortion/miscarriage means that the miscarriage is accompanied by infection inside the uterus.

The last four conditions are discussed further in Chapter 4.

Induced abortion/termination of pregnancy means that the pregnancy was terminated intentionally.

Recurrent miscarriage/abortion is a term usually used to mean that a woman has had three or more consecutive miscarriages; this problem is discussed further in Chapter 9.

2 Ovulation, conception, and early development of the embryo

....

In order to understand more about why miscarriages occur, it is important to know something about the physiology of reproduction, which is discussed in this chapter.

The female reproductive organs consist of the ovaries, fallopian tubes, uterus (womb), cervix (neck of the womb), and vagina as shown in Figure 1.

In a woman of reproductive age, each of the two ovaries is almond-shaped and approximately 3 cm × 1.5 cm × 1 cm in size. Each ovary contains several thousand tiny ovarian follicles, which were all formed when the woman herself was a fetus. Each follicle consists of an immature ovum (egg) surrounded by layers of smaller cells. The fallopian tubes are joined into the uterus and are approximately 10 cm long. The part of each tube that is nearest the uterus is very narrow, whereas the part nearest the ovary (the ampulla) is wider. Fertilization normally takes place in the ampulla. The outer end of each tube is formed of several tentacle-like processes, known as fimbriae, which help the ovum enter the tube at the time of ovulation.

The uterus varies in size from one woman to another. In a woman of reproductive age who has not borne children it is usually approximately 8 cm long, 5 cm wide at its widest point, and 3 cm from front to back. It has a thick muscular wall. The upper part of the uterus is known as the body of the uterus; it is lined with tissue known as the endometrium, most of which is shed with each menstrual period. The body of the uterus is usually tilted forwards (anteverted), but in about one sixth of women it is tilted backwards (retroverted). This is usually of no significance and does not make miscarriage more likely.

The lower part of the uterus is known as the cervix. It protrudes into the top of the vagina, and can be felt by inserting a finger into

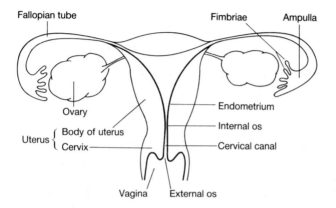

Figure 1 The female reproductive organs.

the vagina. It feels rather like the tip of your nose. Its vaginal surface is normally covered with smooth pink tissue. The inner area of the junction of the body of the uterus and the cervix is known as the internal os. The opening from the lower end of the cervical canal into the vagina is called the external os, which is the area from which cervical smears are taken.

Ovulation

The processes of ovulation and menstruation are controlled by a complicated interplay between the pituitary gland and the ovaries (Figure 2). The pituitary gland is only about 1 cm in diameter but it is a very important structure indeed. It lies near the middle of the skull under the lower surface of the brain, and it exerts control over several organs (including the thyroid gland, the adrenal glands, the ovaries, and the testes) by producing various hormones. Hormones are chemical messengers produced in one part of the body which affect the function of cells in other parts of the body. The pituitary hormones that affect the function of the ovaries are known as follicle-stimulating hormone (FSH) and luteinizing hormone (LH). Other hormones which affect the baby's development, the labour, and the birth come into play during pregnancy.

Pituitary gland

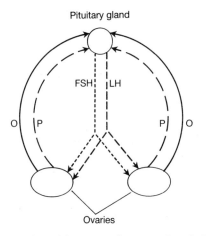

Ovaries

Figure 2 The interplay of hormones between the pituitary gland and the ovaries: FSH, follicle-stimulating hormone; LH, luteinizing hormone; O, oestrogen; P, progesterone.

The average menstrual cycle is approximately 28 days in length. It begins on the first day of a menstrual period and lasts until the next period starts. The first half of the cycle, leading up to ovulation, is known as the follicular phase; the second half of the cycle (after ovulation) is known as the luteal phase (Figure 3). The luteal phase usually lasts from 10 to 14 days. The follicular phase is more variable in length; it lasts about 14 days in an average cycle but is much longer in some women. Thus in a woman with a 35 day cycle the follicular phase lasts approximately 21 days.

During the follicular phase, several of the many follicles present in the ovaries increase in size under the influence of the follicle-stimulating hormone (FSH) produced by the pituitary gland. One follicle usually develops faster than the others and becomes the 'dominant follicle'. As the follicles develop, they secrete increasing amounts of oestrogen (one of the two sorts of female hormone) which causes regrowth of the endometrial lining of the uterus. The increasing oestrogen levels also affect the production and secretion of other hormones by the pituitary gland, leading to a greatly increased release or 'surge' of luteinizing hormone (LH)

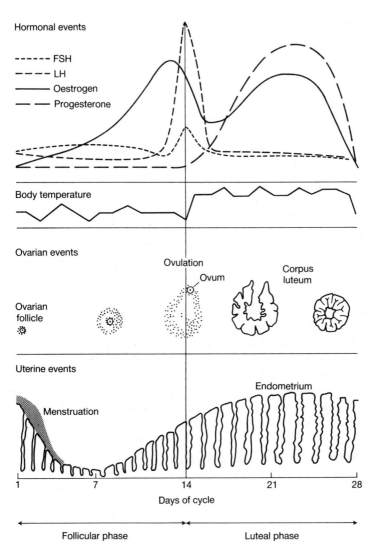

Figure 3 The events of the normal menstrual cycle: FSH, follicle-stimulating hormone; LH, luteinizing hormone.

on about day 12 or 13 of a normal cycle. This causes ovulation to occur approximately 24 hours later from the fully developed dominant follicle, which by then is about the size of a small tomato (approximately 2 cm diameter). Sometimes ovulation will occur from more than one mature follicle.

The fimbriae (tentacles) of the fallopian tube become closely applied to the ovary during ovulation, and the ovum and its surrounding cells are guided along the fallopian tube by the action of millions of cilia (hair-like processes) on the cells lining the tube, and by the contractions of the tube.

Following ovulation the ovarian follicle collapses and develops into a corpus luteum, or 'yellow body', so called because of its yellowish colour (Figure 3). The corpus luteum secretes increasing amounts of progesterone (the other female hormone) and also continues to produce oestrogens. Under the influence of progesterone, there is further development of the endometrium in the luteal phase in preparation for the arrival of a fertilized ovum. If implantation (embedding) of an ovum does not follow, oestrogen and progesterone levels fall, the endometrium disintegrates, and a menstrual period occurs with loss of blood and endometrial tissue (Figure 3). If implantation of a fertilized ovum does occur, the corpus luteum continues to secrete increasing amounts of oestrogen and progesterone during the early weeks of pregnancy. The rise in progesterone levels in the luteal phase is responsible for the slight rise in body temperature (approximately 0.5°F or 0.3°C) that occurs after ovulation (Figure 3). Measurement of the body temperature (first thing in the morning) during two or three cycles is helpful in showing whether a progesterone-producing corpus luteum has formed, and thus whether ovulation has presumably occurred. However, it is not a useful way of timing intercourse to coincide with ovulation in a particular cycle, as the temperature rise may not be clear cut, and by the time that a persistent rise in the temperature has occurred it may be too late for fertilization to take place.

Sperm production

Sperms are produced in large numbers in the testes and are stored in the male reproductive tract prior to ejaculation. Each ejaculate contains several million sperms, which are deposited high in the vagina during intercourse. Many of them rapidly penetrate the cervical mucus, which is receptive to them around the time of ovulation, although not at other times in the cycle. The sperms then pass into the uterus and along the fallopian tubes, which some of them reach within minutes of ejaculation. Their numbers decline markedly within 24 hours of intercourse, but a few may remain in the fallopian tubes and retain their ability to fertilize for more than 48 hours.

Fertilization

Fertilization of an ovum by a sperm normally takes place in the ampulla of one of the fallopian tubes; it is only possible for a few hours after ovulation. It is a highly complex process which has become better understood in recent years. It is at this time that many fetal chromosomal abnormalities arise; others arise during the earlier development of either the ovum or the sperm.

At the time of fertilization each ovum or sperm contains half the number of chromosomes that are present in other cells, so that when they fuse the fertilized ovum will have the normal complement of 46 chromosomes comprised of 23 pairs. One pair of chromosomes determines the sex of the person (Plate 1). In a female both the sex chromosomes are so-called 'X' chromosomes; in a male there is one 'X' chromosome and one 'Y' chromosome in each cell. The chromosomes are made up of thousands of genes which transmit all the information necessary to create a human being with characteristics (such as height, hair colour, blood group etc.) inherited from both parents.

Thus each ovum has 22 non-sex chromosomes and an X chromosome, and each sperm has 22 non-sex chromosomes and either an X or a Y chromosome. If the fertilizing sperm bears an X chromosome, the fertilized ovum and all the cells into which it divides will contain two X chromosomes, and the fetus will develop as a female. If the fertilizing sperm bears a Y chromosome, the fetus will develop as a male.

Producing the right number of complete chromosomes is more complicated than it may sound. It is not a simple division of the chromosomes, with one member of each pair going into each ovum or sperm. When ova and sperm are created, there is an exchange of chromosomal material between the members of each pair of chromosomes before half the parental chromosomal material becomes part of the new ovum or sperm. This allows for great variety in the genetic make-up of each individual ovum and sperm, and hence of each individual human being.

The process of exchanging and integrating the chromosomal material of the ovum and the sperm at the time of fertilization is also highly complicated. It is not surprising, therefore, that errors in the chromosomal make-up of the fertilized ovum commonly occur. Sometimes the chromosomes are damaged when they exchange material and sometimes the egg or sperm ends up with too many or too few chromosomes. It is thought that such errors arise in more than half of all conceptions. In the great majority of these cases the chromosomal abnormality is so severe that the embryo dies during the early days or weeks of pregnancy, often before the woman knows that she is pregnant. It has been found that a chromosomal abnormality is present in more than half of confirmed pregnancies which end in miscarriage (see Chapter 7).

The chromosomes of an adult or child can be studied by culturing white blood cells from a blood sample, in a specialized laboratory, and then making a detailed examination of the chromosomes. Fetal chromosomes can be studied by culturing a sample of amniotic fluid (the fluid surrounding the fetus), taken by amniocentesis, or by examining a sample of placental tissue taken by chorionic villus sampling (CVS) or occasionally by examination of fetal blood obtained by cordocentesis (see Chapter 11).

Implantation

The fertilized ovum begins to divide as it moves along the fallopian tube towards the uterus. Its movement is caused by the beating of the cilia and by the muscular contractions of the tube. It enters the uterus after it has divided into eight or more cells, about 3 or 4 days after fertilization. Cell division continues before the ovum implants (embeds) in the suitably prepared endometrium, about 6 or 7 days after fertilization, at which stage it is still smaller than a pin head.

The process of implantation is very complex, and not surprisingly many fertilized ova fail to implant satisfactorily and are lost at this time. Soon after implantation, increasing amounts of a hormone known as human chorionic gonadotrophin (hCG) are made by the microscopic projections of the placenta known as chorionic villi. Detection of hCG forms the basis of the standard pregnancy test on an early morning urine sample, as its production is almost unique to pregnancy. Very low levels of this hormone can now be measured in blood and urine, and so-called 'subclinical' pregnancies can be detected before a menstrual period has been missed, less than 14 days after fertilization. From studies involving such measurements of hCG in women trying to conceive, it appears that between one-tenth and one-third of embryos are lost during the second week after fertilization, without the women being aware that they had been pregnant (see Chapter 6).

Further growth of the embryo

Following successful implantation further rapid growth and development of the embryo take place. The embryo is very vulnerable to the effects of harmful agents such as certain infections, for example rubella (German measles), and some drugs, as the various organs develop. This is why it is important that women should have their immunity to rubella confirmed before they become pregnant, and why X-ray examinations and most drugs should be avoided when conception is a possibility.

However, chromosome abnormalities occur much more commonly than abnormalities due to harmful agents; the latter are sometimes avoidable, while chromosome abnormalities are not.

3 *Threatened miscarriage and ectopic pregnancy*

● ●

Vaginal bleeding in early pregnancy is a very common problem. It probably occurs in about 1 in 4 confirmed pregnancies. In many cases the bleeding is slight and settles down, and the source is never identified with certainty. The bleeding may come from inside the uterus and be due to a complication of pregnancy such as a threatened or actual miscarriage, or it can be related to an ectopic pregnancy (pregnancy in one of the fallopian tubes), or it may come from the cervix. Bleeding in early pregnancy comes from the mother and not from the fetus.

Threatened miscarriage

The main symptom of a threatened miscarriage is bleeding from the vagina which is usually red to start with, and then changes to brown as the amount of loss decreases. It is due to some degree of separation of the placenta or membranes from the wall of the uterus. There may be some lower abdominal discomfort and backache, similar to that felt with a menstrual period. Often the bleeding stops after a few hours or days, but it may stop and start over several weeks, with the pregnancy still continuing normally. In some cases, however, the fetus will die before or after the bleeding has started, and a miscarriage will eventually take place.

If the bleeding becomes heavy with clots or if the pain becomes severe, it is likely that a miscarriage is occurring and the general practitioner should be contacted. Any tissue that is passed should be kept so that it can be checked by the doctor and if necessary sent for examination under a microscope.

Diagnosis of threatened miscarriage

The doctor may perform an internal examination in order to distinguish between a threatened and an actual miscarriage. With a threatened miscarriage, the uterus is the appropriate size for the length of gestation and the cervical canal is 'closed' (its normal diameter). If a miscarriage has already occurred, the placental tissue and amniotic sac, which may contain a fetus, may have been only partially expelled. They may be lying partly in the uterus and partly in the cervical canal and the vagina; this is known as an incomplete miscarriage. If all the tissue has been expelled the uterus will have become smaller and the cervical canal will have become 'closed' again (Figure 1).

If a diagnosis of threatened miscarriage is made, an ultrasound scan (Plate 2) will probably be arranged to confirm that the fetus is alive and to exclude the unlikely possibility of a hydatidiform mole (see Chapter 7). If it is not possible for this to be done, a pregnancy test may be performed, but this can remain positive even after the fetus has died as the placenta may continue to make human chorionic gonadotrophin (hCG), and it takes some days for hCG to be cleared from the body.

Many hospitals now have Early Pregnancy Units where women

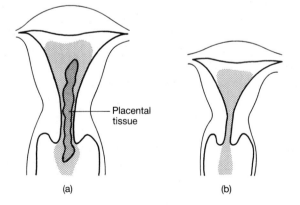

(a)   (b)

Figure 1 (a) Incomplete miscarriage; (b) complete miscarriage.

with bleeding or pain in early pregnancy can be scanned within a day or two of the onset of symptoms so that a diagnosis of threatened miscarriage, incomplete or complete miscarriage, or ectopic pregnancy can be made and appropriate advice can be given. By 7 weeks from the beginning of the last menstrual period (5 weeks after conception) the fetus should be easily visible by ultrasound in the amniotic sac within the uterus and the fetal heart should be seen to be beating.

Treatment of threatened miscarriage

It is very difficult to prove that any particular treatment reduces the chance that a threatened miscarriage will proceed to a miscarriage. In many cases the pregnancy will continue normally without any special action being taken; in other cases the fetus will already have died and nothing can be done to save it.

The two general measures which seem most likely to be beneficial for a precarious pregnancy, and which are most often recommended, are resting and refraining from sexual intercourse. Rest is interpreted by different people in different ways. In general, if the abdominal discomfort and bleeding are slight then it may not be important for the woman to stay in bed. If, however, there is fairly heavy bleeding bed rest may lessen the amount of bleeding, and it may also reduce the chance of miscarriage. It is hard to prove that it helps, but it is possible that it may make all the difference in a few cases.

The reasoning behind avoiding sexual intercourse is that the uterus contracts during orgasm, and if the pregnancy is already in danger of being expelled the contractions may be sufficient to precipitate a miscarriage. Another danger of intercourse is the possibility that infection may be introduced into the uterus if a miscarriage has already begun.

Drug and hormone treatment of threatened miscarriage

A large number of remedies have been tried, but there is no evidence that any drugs or hormones have any beneficial effects at all; indeed some of them actually have short-term, or more often long-term, ill effects.

Short-term ill effects include prolonging the time to spontaneous miscarriage when the fetus has already died. This may occur with some progestogens (progesterone and progesterone-like drugs).

The main long-term worry with drugs and hormones is that they may harm the fetus. This effect may be apparent when the baby is born; thus thalidomide caused severe limb deformities, and some progestogens used in the past caused masculinization of some female fetuses. Or it may not be apparent for many years; thus some years ago it was found that some of the daughters of women who were given diethylstilboestrol (DES, a synthetic oestrogen) in pregnancy, mainly in the 1950s, have an abnormally developed uterus and are also at risk for developing a rare type of vaginal cancer in their teens and early twenties. Stilboestrol is no longer given to pregnant women.

Sedatives

Sympathetic explanation and reassurance are preferable to the administration of sedatives which cannot help to save the pregnancy and which may even be harmful.

Analgesics (pain-relieving drugs)

Severe pain does not usually occur with a threatened miscarriage; if pain is continuous or severe a doctor should be consulted. It is likely that a miscarriage is occurring or, much less commonly, that the pregnancy is in one of the fallopian tubes (ectopic pregnancy) instead of in the uterus (see p. 16).

Hormones

There is no definite evidence that any miscarriages are due to inadequate production of any particular hormone. Low hormone levels may sometimes be found prior to miscarriage, but this is usually because the pregnancy has already failed; the low levels are not usually the cause of the failure.

Hormones that are still occasionally used in an attempt to support an early pregnancy include hCG, progesterone, and non-masculinizing progestogens. There is no evidence that any of these are effective, although it is possible that they may be in a very few cases. Hormonal treatment, which can sometimes cause problems, is therefore seldom justified except in some forms of assisted conception treatment where hormones may need to be given to support an early pregnancy.

Outlook for the pregnancy following a threatened miscarriage

The outlook for the pregnancy following a threatened miscarriage is very good if the bleeding settles and the fetus is still alive. Thus in more than nine out of ten such cases the pregnancy will end with the birth of a live healthy baby. Many women are anxious that there may be a greatly increased risk of their baby being abnormal when they have had bleeding in early pregnancy, but fortunately this is not so. There is, however, a slightly increased risk of premature labour and of impaired placental function later in pregnancy, and it is therefore important that the pregnancy should be carefully monitored with these problems in mind.

Ectopic pregnancy

If the abdominal pain is very severe or unrelenting the possibility of an ectopic pregnancy must be considered. This is a potentially very dangerous condition as internal bleeding occurs and this can lead to collapse and even to death if an emergency operation is not performed in time (see p. 17). Ectopic means out of place, and the term ectopic pregnancy is used to describe a pregnancy that has implanted outside the uterine cavity. This occurs in about 1 in 100 pregnancies in Britain. The number of ectopic pregnancies is increasing, partly because they are commoner in women who undergo assisted conception treatment. The most common site for an ectopic pregnancy is in one of the fallopian tubes. As the pregnancy develops the tube stretches and may rupture (Figure 2).

If the pregnancy implants in the narrow part of the tube, rupture of the tube and internal haemorrhage leading to severe abdominal pain, faintness, and collapse are likely to occur very early in the pregnancy, sometimes before the woman knows that she is pregnant. More commonly, an ectopic pregnancy implants in the wider part of the tube (the ampulla) and internal bleeding then

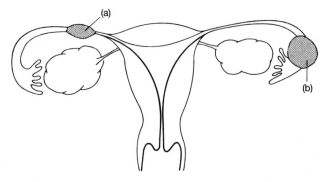

Figure 2 Two common sites for an ectopic pregnancy: (a) in the narrow part of the fallopian tube; (b) in the wider part of the fallopian tube (ampulla).

occurs a little later in the first trimester and will often be less dramatic, so that the abdominal pain may be less sudden in onset and less severe. There is often some vaginal bleeding.

The diagnosis may be difficult to make, but the important thing is that it should be considered. When the diagnosis is obvious, an emergency abdominal operation under general anaesthesia is required and the affected tube will often have to be removed as it will be so damaged. A blood transfusion may be needed to replace the blood lost into the abdominal cavity.

If the diagnosis is uncertain, a laparoscopy will often be recommended. In this procedure (which is usually done under general anaesthesia) a pencil-sized lighted telescope (laparoscope) is inserted just under the umbilicus (navel), after filling the abdominal cavity with carbon dioxide, and a good view of the uterus, fallopian tubes, and ovaries can be obtained. If the diagnosis of ectopic pregnancy is confirmed, the gynaecologist will proceed straightaway to operate on the affected tube. This is increasingly done using a laparoscopic technique. Sometimes the tube can be saved.

The quality of ultrasound images is improving all the time, and is much better in early pregnancy when the scan is performed using a transvaginal probe (which is inserted into the vagina) than when it is performed via the abdomen using a standard transabdominal probe.

The diagnosis of ectopic pregnancy is being made earlier and earlier in pregnancy. It can be made before a woman has any symptoms, if the woman has a reason to be scanned in early pregnancy, for example if she has undergone assisted conception, or if she has had a previous ectopic pregnancy or more than one miscarriage.

In some centres early ectopic pregnancies are injected under ultrasound or laparoscopic control to prevent them developing further and an operation may then be unnecessary. The fallopian tube can thus be saved and will often function normally.

Outlook for the future following an ectopic pregnancy

Although the risk of having an ectopic pregnancy is increased in a woman who has already had an ectopic pregnancy, there is a good chance, if she becomes pregnant again, that her next pregnancy will be in the womb and that it will proceed normally. It will be important for her to have an early scan when she becomes pregnant again, to determine whether the pregnancy is indeed in the womb.

Other causes of bleeding in early pregnancy

Bleeding in early pregnancy may be due to complications of pregnancy as described above or it may be due to other causes such as a cervical ectropion, a cervical polyp, or very rarely cancer of the cervix.

Cervical ectropion

This term is used to describe a change in the cervix which commonly occurs during pregnancy and at other times of hormonal change (such as when a woman is taking a hormonal contraceptive pill). The cervical canal is normally lined by mucus-producing cells which make it look red and rough to the naked eye, whereas the vaginal surface of the cervix (the ectocervix) normally appears pink and smooth (Figure 3). With the alteration in hormone levels that occurs in pregnancy, the red mucus-producing tissue lining the cervical canal is exposed by a slight gaping of the cervix and the ectocervix appears red and rough. This appearance is known

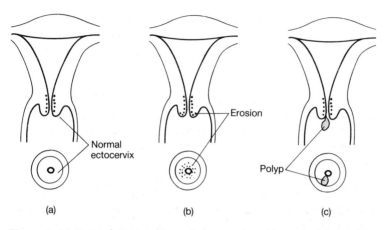

Figure 3 (a) Normal cervix; (b) cervical ectropion; (c) cervical polyp. The appearance of the cervix on speculum examination is shown in the lower part of the diagram.

as a cervical ectropion (Figure 3). (It was previously inappropriately called an 'erosion', although the cervix is not in fact eroded.)

The mucus-producing tissue is more fragile and bleeds more readily than the pink smooth tissue which usually covers the ectocervix. It is not uncommon for bleeding to occur after intercourse, or even spontaneously, when a cervical ectropion is present. Provided that a cervical smear is normal, a cervical ectropion should be left untreated during pregnancy. It will usually disappear in the weeks following delivery.

Cervical polyp

Another less common condition which may cause bleeding in early pregnancy is a cervical polyp (Figure 3). This is a benign (non-malignant) roughly spherical growth on a stalk that arises from the cervical canal. Polyps vary in size from a few millimetres to over a centimetre in diameter. They are covered in red mucus-producing tissue and may bleed spontaneously or when touched. They should be left alone during pregnancy and no attempt should be made to remove them as this may cause undue bleeding. They are usually found to have disappeared when the cervix is examined at the postnatal check up (approximately six weeks after delivery).

Cancer of the cervix

Although less than 1 in 1000 women who have bleeding in early pregnancy will be found to have cancer of the cervix, it is important that anyone with persistent vaginal bleeding should have an internal examination so that the cervix can be looked at and a cervical smear can be taken if appropriate.

In summary, bleeding from the vagina in early pregnancy is a common problem. In many cases it will settle without treatment and the pregnancy will continue normally. In some cases, however, the bleeding will herald the onset of a miscarriage, or it may be indicative of a different problem such as an ectopic pregnancy or a cervical abnormality.

• •

I became pregnant the first month after my husband and I decided to try to have children. I was doing very vigorous exercise at the time and did not realise at first that I was pregnant, as I did not miss a period. I had a miscarriage at 6 weeks but it took two months for the bleeding to stop and at one point I thought I had had two miscarriages in quick succession. I was surprised at how upset I felt—somehow I felt a bit of a failure and guilty that the exercise had caused the miscarriage. At the back of my mind I wondered if I would ever be able to have children.

I had a very reassuring consultation with the author and tried to stop worrying and to relax. Five months later I became pregnant again when I was feeling particularly relaxed and happy, as I was in the last two weeks of a job that I hated.

I was very careful during my pregnancy—I had a lot of rest, no alcohol, and no heavy lifting—and I had a completely straightforward pregnancy culminating in an incredibly short and easy labour and a healthy 9 lb 6 oz boy! In retrospect my miscarriage was probably a good thing as it made me appreciate that life is a gift and it made having a child seem extra special.

• •

4 Complete and incomplete miscarriage; missed abortion

The first warning that a pregnancy may end in a miscarriage is usually the occurrence of vaginal bleeding. In many cases, as discussed in the last chapter, vaginal bleeding in early pregnancy will stop and will not be followed by a miscarriage. Unfortunately, however, in some cases a miscarriage will take place. Usually the bleeding becomes heavier and painful uterine contractions occur. The pain is usually intermittent, coming every few minutes, as in labour. The amount of pain experienced differs from one woman to another, and in the same woman from one pregnancy to another, as does the time taken for a miscarriage to occur after the contractions have begun. This can vary from minutes to several hours. If the pain is severe and the woman is in hospital, a pain-killing injection can be given, provided that the possibility of an ectopic pregnancy has been excluded.

As the bleeding increases, blood clots and placental tissue and membranes may be passed. In early pregnancy, if the fetus has died some time before the miscarriage occurs, it may have dissolved away and no longer be identifiable. Later in pregnancy, a recognizable fetus may be present. Any tissue that is passed should be saved for the doctor to examine. This examination is important for several reasons. Firstly, if recognizable placental tissue has been expelled, a certain diagnosis of actual rather than threatened miscarriage can be made, and it may be possible to tell whether the miscarriage is complete or incomplete. Secondly, the presence of recognizable placental tissue will give proof that the woman was definitely pregnant. It is possible for there to be a delayed menstrual period followed by very heavy bleeding and the passage of blood clots without a woman being pregnant, and it can be very important for her future to know whether or not she was pregnant; if, for example, there are questions about the couple's fertility and the pregnancy is confirmed, it will be clear that there was no bar to conception on this occasion. Thirdly, examination of the tissue may occasionally help to explain why the miscarriage occurred.

Complete miscarriage

With a complete miscarriage all the tissue is expelled from the uterus, which is then empty, and a curettage (scrape) is not required. The vaginal bleeding will become progressively less in amount and should cease after a few days. Very early miscarriages, before 7 weeks' gestation, are usually complete (Figure 1).

Incomplete miscarriage

Later miscarriages are, unfortunately, often incomplete and some pieces of placental tissue may remain inside the uterus. This is a potentially dangerous situation as heavy bleeding may occur, and there is also a risk that the tissue will become infected in due course. It is therefore important that medical advice should be sought if there is a possibility that a miscarriage is incomplete.

Heavy bleeding may occur because there is a very good blood supply to the uterus and placenta throughout pregnancy. With a miscarriage, the placenta separates from the wall of the uterus and the maternal blood vessels are then exposed and are able to bleed. If all the tissue is expelled, the muscle fibres in the wall of the uterus can contract and close off the exposed vessels. If, however, tissue is retained in the uterus, the muscle fibres are unable to contract fully and heavy bleeding may ensue. Fortunately there are drugs available (such as ergometrine and syntocinon) which make the muscle fibres contract more efficiently, and the amount of bleeding can usually be temporarily reduced by the administration of one or both of these drugs. However, the only way to ensure that heavy bleeding does not recur is for the uterus to be emptied. This has to be done in hospital. If the bleeding is severe, it may be necessary to give a blood transfusion before or during the procedure. Rarely, if a woman has a very heavy blood loss she will need to be resuscitated with an intravenous infusion (drip), and blood if necessary, before she is taken to hospital.

As a general anaesthetic is usually required to allow the uterus to be emptied, nothing should be eaten or drunk while awaiting transfer to hospital following a miscarriage. An empty stomach is needed to reduce the risk of vomiting and inhalation of the stomach contents into the lungs during the operation. If there is an urgent need to give an anaesthetic before the stomach is empty, the anaesthetist will usually insert a cuffed endotracheal tube into the trachea (windpipe), after putting the woman to sleep, to reduce the risk of such inhalation. Under anaesthetic, the uterus is gently emptied of any remaining tissue. An injection of ergometrine or syntocinon is often given to encourage the uterus to contract and to reduce the blood loss. After the operation there should be no pain other than the discomfort, like a period pain, caused by the contractions of the uterus; the amount of bleeding will be similar to that which occurs during a normal period. The nurses will check the pulse and blood pressure, and the blood loss for some time after the procedure. Once they are satisfied that the woman's condition is stable and that she is properly 'round' from the anaesthetic and not nauseated, she will be able to eat and drink, and to get up and about. If she is Rhesus-negative she should receive an injection of anti-D to minimize the likelihood of developing anti-Rhesus positive (D) antibodies (see page 59). Practices vary and she may go home the same day or stay over night after the operation.

Sometimes the breasts will become uncomfortable and start leaking milk after a miscarriage. The later in pregnancy that a miscarriage occurs, the more likely is this to happen. Provided that the milk is not expressed (squeezed out) the breasts will usually stop leaking, without any special treatment, but occasionally drug treatment will be needed.

It is normal for a deep sense of loss to be experienced following a miscarriage; this is discussed further in the next chapter (Chapter 5).

Loss of one of twins in early pregnancy

It is possible for twins to be conceived, for one twin to die in early pregnancy, and for the other twin to continue to develop normally. Twenty years ago it was thought that this occurred quite often, but it has now been realised that the early ultrasound diagnosis of twins was frequently incorrect. A clear area outside the sac was often interpreted as being a second sac, when it was just a collection of fluid or blood. It has now been realised that ultrasound diagnosis of twin pregnancy should not be made until two hearts can be seen to be beating (at about 7 weeks' gestation). If one twin does die in early pregnancy, the chance of the remaining twin surviving to term is good.

Septic abortion/miscarriage

Fortunately, infection does not usually occur following a spontaneous miscarriage if the uterus is emptied at the time of, or within a few hours of, the miscarriage. However, infection can arise at any time and if it does prompt treatment is important as otherwise the infection may ascend from the uterus to the fallopian tubes and cause salpingitis (inflammation of the fallopian tubes). This can lead, in a small percentage of cases, to permanent damage of the fallopian tubes and to subsequent infertility. Another danger is that occasionally the infection can spread beyond the fallopian tubes into the abdominal (peritoneal) cavity, causing peritonitis and a severe generalized illness.

If infection does occur, modern antibiotics can usually bring it rapidly under control. It is essential, however, that an adequate course of the appropriate antibiotics is completed to ensure that the infection is completely eliminated.

Missed abortion/miscarriage (early embryonic loss)

These terms are used to describe the situation that can arise when a fetus dies but the pregnancy is not expelled. It is 'missed' in the sense that a miscarriage has not occurred, rather than that it has occurred without anyone noticing. Initially the woman will be unaware that anything is wrong, but then she may notice that her pregnancy symptoms are subsiding and that she no longer feels pregnant. There may be some vaginal bleeding. If a vaginal examination is performed the uterus will usually be found to be smaller than the size expected for the known length of pregnancy.

The best method of confirming or refuting a diagnosis of missed abortion is to perform an ultrasound scan. If the fetus is alive the fetal heart can usually be seen to be beating by 7 weeks from the last menstrual period (5 weeks after conception). By about 12 weeks' gestation it should be possible to hear the fetal heart sounds using a portable doppler ultrasound machine, which is a much simpler piece of apparatus than an ultrasound scanner. The probe is placed on the lower abdomen and the woman will be able to hear the fetal heart sounds too, if they are present, and this will obviously be very reassuring. In early pregnancy it will sometimes be necessary to perform more than one ultrasound scan before a diagnosis of missed abortion can be made or excluded with certainty. A pregnancy test is less helpful than an ultrasound scan because, as mentioned previously, it can remain positive for some days after the fetus has died.

It is very distressing for a woman to know that she is carrying a fetus which is no longer alive, and for this reason many women will be anxious to have the uterus emptied as soon as possible once the diagnosis of missed abortion is certain. Such a course of action will also spare the woman some of the trauma of a spontaneous miscarriage. It is extremely important, however, to be quite sure of the diagnosis before the uterus is emptied. The only medical danger in not emptying the uterus promptly is that occasionally changes will occur in the mother's blood, a few weeks after the fetus has died, which may make it clot less well, which could result in heavy bleeding when the miscarriage finally takes place. These changes can be tested for, and if necessary treatment with the appropriate clotting factors can be given.

Nowadays the uterus can either be emptied surgically, as described under 'Incomplete miscarriage' (page 23) or occasionally by using medication. Medication usually consists of mifepristone which is taken by mouth in hospital. The woman then goes home for about 48 hours and returns to the hospital in order to be given a prostaglandin pessary, which is inserted into the vagina. This treatment will usually cause a miscarriage to occur; it is relatively new and is not yet widely available.

Continued bleeding following a miscarriage

If heavy bleeding continues following a miscarriage, it is likely that some tissue is still present in the uterus or that infection has occurred. Curettage and/or treatment with antibiotics may be necessary.

Advice following a miscarriage

Because of the danger of introducing infection, it is wise not to use tampons for the bleeding that occurs after a miscarriage, and not to resume intercourse for at least two weeks. Many women will prefer to wait to have intercourse until after they have had a period. It is common for couples to find that their sex drive is reduced for a while after a miscarriage.

The normal menstrual cycle usually recommences soon after a miscarriage, and a period commonly occurs within four to six weeks. This is usually preceded by ovulation, and so if a couple wish to have intercourse without conceiving for a while, some form of contraception should be used. If contraceptive pills are preferred, they can be started the day after the miscarriage occurred. Extra precautions (such as condoms) should, as usual, be used during the first month. It is generally advisable to wait two or three months before trying for another pregnancy, but there is no known risk associated with becoming pregnant again straight away. A delay of a few months allows for physical and emotional adjustment but is not essential. It used to be helpful to allow a regular cycle to resume before becoming pregnant so that the next pregnancy could be dated accurately, to allow optimum management, but with the advent of ultrasound scans this is no longer so important.

Outlook for the future

The likelihood of having a healthy baby in another pregnancy following a miscarriage will obviously depend on the reason why the miscarriage occurred. However, in statistical terms, if a woman's first pregnancy ends in the first three months of pregnancy she is probably only very slightly more at risk of a miscarriage in her second pregnancy than someone of the same age and background who has had no miscarriages. Following two consecutive miscarriages, the chance of the next confirmed pregnancy ending in the birth of a live healthy baby is still about 7 out of 10 (70 %), and even after three miscarriages it is greater than 5 out of 10 (50 %). None the less, if a woman has three or more consecutive miscarriages it may be helpful to consider undertaking some special tests (see Chapter 9). Advice on precautions to be taken in a pregnancy which follows a miscarriage is given in Chapter 10.

• •

Nearly four years ago a home testing kit confirmed that I was pregnant but as the next couple of weeks passed I felt rather uneasy as I experienced only very transient symptoms of nausea and breast tenderness. Slight bleeding began at around seven weeks and a few days later I realised that I had not felt any symptoms of pregnancy for several days. About ten days after the bleeding started it became much heavier and I began to experience dragging pains and eventually stomach cramps. I was sent to a hospital where I was told that the cervix was still closed and that an ultrasound was required to determine what was happening. This was booked for four days later. I returned to the hospital again during the weekend and although I was told that the pregnancy might still be all right I found this difficult to believe since the pain was by now very intense and the bleeding very heavy. The miscarriage occurred on the Monday (at 9 1/2 weeks) after which I felt quite shocked for a couple of hours. Firstly because I had not expected the pain to be so great and secondly because I was quite unprepared for the fetal form to be so clearly distinguishable, and I found this extremely upsetting. Feelings of shock were then replaced by an overwhelming sense of emptiness. Although I had tried very hard to be philosophical, and I knew that I was lucky to have conceived very quickly, I still felt indescribably sad. An ultrasound was carried out on the Wednesday and I was told that a D and C would not be necessary and that I should wait for three months and then try again. I found the medical staff very flippant on this occasion, and on the day that the miscarriage occurred, and I felt very angry about this for some time as well as feeling emotional about the loss.

My next pregnancy was confirmed a few months later and, although friends and relatives considered I was acting neurotically, I again felt convinced that my symptoms were rather erratic. Eventually I stopped discussing this as people always countered my concerns with 'it wouldn't happen twice'. I reached 8 weeks uneventfully and wondered if I was not just being overly pessimistic. However, at 10 weeks I started to bleed and events then followed a very similar pattern to those that had occurred previously. I went to my general practitioner who confirmed that the cervix was still closed but she explained that she could not predict what might happen and that no medical intervention could actually stop a miscarriage occurring at this stage. A couple of days later I woke in the early hours of the morning, in a lot of pain, and at least this time I recognized what was happening. I was 11 ½ weeks pregnant by this time. I felt less shocked than on the previous occasion but rather more upset, since the pregnancy was expelled in two distinct stages with a six hour interval in between and I thought perhaps it had been a twin pregnancy, which made me feel even more emotional. This time I was admitted to a different hospital and a D and C was performed. Rather illogically I felt more positive at this stage than I had six months earlier; I think this was due to the sensitive approach of the medical and nursing staff at this hospital and the knowledge that if I became pregnant again I would be followed more closely.

We made a concerted effort to concentrate on aspects of our lives other than starting a family and in fact it was six months before I felt that I would like to be pregnant again. My third pregnancy was confirmed towards the end of the year and this time there was reason to feel more hopeful; my ultrasound at 6 ½ weeks showed that the heart beat was already present and I felt my symptoms were strong and constant. Some bleeding occurred again at 8 weeks but this time it lasted only a few days and a healthy baby boy was born at term. I then had another straightforward pregnancy with the birth of a second healthy baby boy, at term, 15 months later.

•••

5 *The emotional effects of miscarriage*

• •

A miscarriage is usually a deeply distressing event to the woman concerned and to those who are closest to her. She, her partner, and her closest relatives and friends are likely to be the people most affected, but obviously circumstances will vary from one woman to another.

The couple will have experienced the joy of achieving a pregnancy and of anticipating the arrival of a baby. Even early in pregnancy the baby may feel very real to them and they may have an image of it in their minds, choose possible names for it, and make extensive plans for its future. As the pregnancy proceeds more relatives and friends will know about it, and more physical preparations for the arrival of the baby will be made such as decorating the nursery and purchasing equipment and even toys. The later in pregnancy that a miscarriage occurs, the greater the parents' distress is likely to be, but an early miscarriage can be equally traumatic, particularly if there was some degree of infertility. Many people are unaware how commonly early miscarriages occur, which means that a miscarriage often comes as a terrible shock.

When a miscarriage occurs, especially in early pregnancy, it may be very difficult for outsiders who have not experienced a similar loss to appreciate the enormity of what has happened to the couple, and to understand that the baby was a very real person to them, with a real identity. The loss of the pregnancy may leave the parents grief-stricken for a considerable period of time. Such lack of understanding may isolate the couple from their acquaintances and make their distress even greater. People may be afraid to talk to them about what has happened as they do not know what to say, as happens with other types of bereavement. With better awareness of the feelings and problems that the couple face some of their suffering can be alleviated. They need people to talk to who can listen and understand. For someone just to say 'Don't worry, you can always try again,' or 'Better luck next time,' ignores the depth of the couple's grief.

Many emotions may be engendered by a miscarriage, and different ones will come to the surface at different times in the days and weeks following the miscarriage. These emotions include fear of the process of miscarriage and about the future, profound disappointment, grief, anger, self-pity, feelings of inadequacy, failure, and helplessness, guilt, jealousy of those who have children, overwhelming sadness and sometimes prolonged depression.

All these feelings may persist for a long time and are easily reawakened by a wide variety of events—particularly by such events as casual contact with pregnant women and children when out shopping, careless remarks by relatives, friends, and acquaintances, photographs and articles in newspapers and magazines, and programmes on the radio or television—or they may just return out of the blue. It is particularly likely that they will be reawakened on the date when the baby was due and on anniversaries of that date, at times of family reunion such as Christmas, and also during a subsequent pregnancy.

The emotions that are felt by the woman and the strength of these emotions will obviously depend on her situation and her previous experiences. All women will be upset to a greater or lesser extent. The pregnancy may even have been unplanned and the woman may have had mixed feelings about it, or have been very upset by it, but even then it is common for her to feel guilty about the miscarriage. She may feel that the fact that she was not pleased about the pregnancy somehow caused the miscarriage to occur.

In the days and weeks following a miscarriage, the couple need support and understanding from family and friends. In addition, support groups (see p. 31) can provide reassurance and help from other people who have had similar experiences.

Fear of the process of miscarriage and about the future

It is very important that the parents receive a clear and sympathetic explanation of what is happening at the time of the miscarriage, and of what is likely to happen in the future, from medical and nursing staff. This may help to reduce the fear and the feelings of inadequacy and guilt, which may well be partly based on misapprehensions. Such help should be sought if it is not forthcoming, as it can make a tremendous difference. Fortunately, medical and nursing staff are becoming more aware of the importance of spending time with women who are having and who have had miscarriages, and of encouraging them to express their fears and other emotions and to ask questions.

Disappointment and grief

The couple should not be afraid to express their feelings. It is normal for someone who has had a miscarriage to feel very strong and often uncontrollable emotions. If the pregnancy was fairly far advanced it may be helpful as part of the grieving process for the couple to see the baby and to know what sex it is, and possibly to have a photograph of it. It is normal practice now for such photographs to be taken for parents who lose a baby later in pregnancy. It may also be helpful to talk to someone who has been through a similar experience. Various support groups have been set up and many couples find them very beneficial, even if they had not previously considered themselves to be 'group people'. The Miscarriage Association has support groups in many areas (see page 84).

Anger, self pity, and feelings of inadequacy, failure, and helplessness

At some stage the couple are likely to feel either anger or self pity, or both these emotions. They will ask themselves: 'Why us?' and they will wonder what they have done to deserve such a misfortune.

They are also likely to experience feelings of inadequacy and helplessness, and to wonder why they have failed to achieve what so many other people appear to achieve without any problems. This feeling of inadequacy may extend to other areas of their lives, resulting in a general loss of confidence.

It may help them a little to realise that miscarriages are extremely common, and that many women who appear to have had problem-free pregnancies have in fact had a miscarriage at some stage. The fact that a pregnancy has occurred means that there is a very good chance that they will have a successful pregnancy in the future.

Guilt

It is normal for the woman to feel that she is in some way responsible for the miscarriage and to go over the events of the preceding days and weeks time and time again in her mind. 'If only . . . ,' she will say to herself. She may worry that she ate or drank the wrong things, took too much exercise or went on too long a journey, that she had intercourse the night before, that she was too anxious, that she was not as happy about the pregnancy as she should have been, that she tripped and fell a few days before the miscarriage, that she is not worthy of being a mother, or about a whole host of other things. She may think that things would have happened differently if she had called the doctor earlier, or if she had seen a different doctor, or had been admitted to a different hospital.

It is very unlikely, however, that any action on her part, or on the part of her medical attendants, was in fact responsible for the miscarriage and she must be encouraged to express her fears so that she can be appropriately reassured. Some people take some comfort from the fact that many miscarriages happen when the fetus is abnormal, and that it would have been even more distressing to have miscarried later in the pregnancy, or to have had an abnormal baby.

In most cases, perhaps fortunately, it will never be known whether the reason for the miscarriage was maternal or paternal, that is whether it was due to a fault in the ovum or the sperm, or some other factor. It is very important that neither the woman nor the man should feel guilty and blame themselves or each other unnecessarily for the miscarriage, and that their families should not do so either. A great deal of distress can be caused by well-intentioned but uninformed comments from relatives and so-called friends. It is natural for people to look for explanations and reasons, but as mentioned elsewhere, it is usually impossible to determine the cause of most miscarriages. Many are due to fetal chromosomal abnormalities, but we do not usually know the cause of these abnormalities.

The father is likely to share some or all of the above feelings. Like the mother, he may feel disappointed, angry, self-pitying, inadequate, helpless, guilty, and depressed. In addition, he will be concerned for the woman's health and safety. He may fear for her life if she is bleeding heavily and has to be admitted to hospital as an emergency. Later he may fear that there will be permanent damage to her (which is very unlikely) and that she may be infertile or that the problem will recur and that they may remain childless.

It is likely that more sympathy and understanding from medical and nursing attendants, and relatives and friends, will be extended to the mother than to the father, and he may feel resentful and left out. It is important, though, for him to feel that his grief is also recognized, even though he may feel that it is unmanly to express his emotions openly. He may try to hide his feelings of disappointment from his partner, thinking that she may become more depressed if she knows how disappointed he is, but if he does this she may think he is insensitive. By keeping his feelings bottled up he may become more depressed later on. He may feel guilty that he was not more helpful with the daily chores during early pregnancy, or that he had to be away on business, or that there is something wrong with his genes.

Men and women express and cope with their feelings in different ways. As in so many other situations good communication and full understanding of each other's feelings are very important and a couple who can share their feelings with each other will obviously be of enormous help and support to one another. It is also important for them to get comfort and support from others as even very strong relationships can suffer from the strain if it is not relieved by family, friends or a support group.

The miscarriage may be the first tragedy that the couple have faced together. Initially sharing the ordeal may bring them closer but later on the stresses that follow may drive them apart. The father may cope with his feelings by not talking about them, while the mother is still grieving openly, and she may think that he is unfeeling and that he does not love her. He may then try to be more supportive but his actions may be misinterpreted. Sexual difficulties commonly occur following a miscarriage and add to the stress. It is important that the couple should be able to discuss their sexual needs with each other.

On the other hand, the couple may be brought closer together and emerge from the crisis with a deeper appreciation of and love for one another. Having come through such an event with their relationship intact or even strengthened should help to boost their confidence in the future.

Effects on children

If there are children in the household it is very likely that they too will be affected by the miscarriage. Even if they have not been told of the pregnancy, they will know that something is wrong, and they will be upset by their parents' obvious or concealed grief. They may feel left out and neglected unless they are allowed to share in their parents' experience. They too may feel guilty and feel that the miscarriage was somehow their fault—if for example they knew that their mother was pregnant and they had been scolded for making her tired or for upsetting her, or for jumping on her, or if they resented the thought of an addition to the family. It should be explained to them, in terms appropriate to their understanding, that the miscarriage was nobody's fault.

••

I had had a normal pregnancy until I was 10 weeks pregnant, when I started bleeding. I had to be admitted to hospital in the middle of the night as I was bleeding heavily and I had a D&C. I never thought that something like this could happen to me: a fit, young, and healthy person. Nobody had warned me how often miscarriages occur. My husband was very shocked and distressed by the miscarriage, too. We did, however, have a lot of support from my family and from friends. I found that I needed to talk about my distress and they listened and this meant that they could understand what we were going through. We were very consoled to learn that people we know have also been through the same upsetting time, more than once for some of them, and that they now have families. It was important for us both to keep busy; working meant that we didn't have too much time to reflect.

I became pregnant again after four months and the early weeks were a time of great anxiety. I had some bleeding at 5 weeks and again at 7 weeks. I had a scan at 8 weeks and it was wonderful to see the pictures and to know that the baby's heart was beating.

My wife's miscarriage was completely unexpected. When it happened I kept saying to myself, 'Why us?'. It didn't seem a fair thing to happen given that a lot of our friends had had babies without any difficulty and knowing how much we wanted a child. I know people who have had problems having babies, but I didn't think that it would be like that for us. I began to wonder what could have caused it—the best that I could come up with was that my wife had been working too hard and I was determined that when she was pregnant again she would not work so hard.

After we started to try again for a child the worrying became worse. The thought that kept going through my mind was, 'Will it happen again?'. We were both very pleased when it was clear that my wife was pregnant again, but I was concerned about the effects that a second miscarriage would have on her. I was worried when she felt unwell in case that was a sign of impending problems; I thought that she was again working too many hours and that this would cause a problem; generally it was a tense time and the weeks passed very slowly. I tried to do as much around the house as possible and to be as supportive as possible. The best moment was when my wife had a scan at 8 weeks and there was actually something there and the heart was beating—it did seem that things were really happening and my fingers remained crossed for the next few weeks.

• •

Happily this couple's second pregnancy continued normally and they were both very relieved when 14 weeks had passed. A scan at 19 weeks showed that the baby was developing normally, and this was very exciting and reassuring. The husband was able to be present for the scan and he felt that at last they could perhaps begin to relax. They were able to have detailed pictures of the baby and this made the baby seem much more real to both of them. The pregnancy continued normally and a healthy baby boy weighing 7 lb 13 oz was delivered at 41 weeks.

6 *The incidence of spontaneous miscarriage*

••

The true incidence of spontaneous miscarriage is very difficult to determine for a variety of reasons. If the term miscarriage is used to include the loss of a fertilized ovum at any stage of its development up to five months or more, it is clear that many 'miscarriages' will occur before a menstrual period has been missed, and thus without the woman ever knowing that she had conceived. Complete miscarriages can also occur after a missed period without the woman realizing that she was pregnant. Even if she was aware that she was pregnant, she may not have been seen by a doctor and the miscarriage may not then be confirmed or recorded. Another problem that can arise is that a woman can miss a period and then have heavy bleeding, and think that she is miscarrying, and yet she may not in fact have been pregnant. It may be difficult to prove whether she was pregnant or not.

Apart from these problems, the frequency of spontaneous miscarriage is likely to vary between different groups of women— for example between those of different ages and different genetic and environmental backgrounds. Nonetheless, through carefully planned surveys and measurements of pregnancy-specific hormone levels in women trying to conceive, knowledge about the true incidence of spontaneous miscarriage has increased. It is clear that the rate of loss is very high in very early pregnancy, and that in general it decreases as pregnancy progresses.

It is difficult to compare miscarriage rates in different countries because of the different definitions used and because miscarriage statistics are often unreliable. Also induced abortions are very common in some countries and this means that the true rate of spontaneous miscarriage is unknown in these countries.

Miscarriages before pregnancy is confirmed

Pre-implantation loss

At the present time it is impossible to know how often an ovum is fertilized and fails to implant (embed) in the uterus, but it is likely that many fail to do so.

Post-implantation loss

After implantation (which occurs about seven days after fertilization) the developing embryo produces increasing amounts of human chorionic gonadotrophin (hCG). Measurement of hCG forms the basis of the standard urinary pregnancy test which usually gives a positive result within a few days after a period is missed. For many pregnancy tests hCG levels have to be relatively high to register, but for research purposes very sensitive assays have been developed which can detect low levels of hCG in the blood or urine, and which can demonstrate the presence of a pregnancy 7–14 days after fertilization. It has been estimated from recent studies using these and other techniques that approximately one in five ova are lost after implantation without the women concerned being aware that they were pregnant.

Miscarriages in confirmed pregnancies

It is somewhat easier to determine the number of pregnancies that are lost after a period has been missed and the woman knows that she is pregnant. It is thought that about 1 in 6 such pregnancies are lost before 14 weeks' gestation (in the first trimester of pregnancy) and that a further 1 in 50 pregnancies are lost during the next 14 weeks (in the second trimester).

In many pregnancies which miscarry the fetus failed to develop normally. If embryonic development ceases at an early stage the amniotic sac may be empty, a condition which used to be referred to as a 'blighted ovum' but which is more appropriately called early embryonic loss or demise. Once a fetal heart beat can be detected, however, the likelihood of a miscarriage is much reduced—to less than 1 in 20.

Risk of miscarriage in women with fertility problems

There seems to be a slightly greater risk of miscarriage in women with decreased fertility than in women who have no difficulty in conceiving, both when they are not receiving any treatment and in some instances when they are receiving treatment. In either case the chance of a pregnancy being successful is still of the order of 7 out of 10 (70%) or more.

The incidence of miscarriage after *in vitro* ('test tube') fertilization, and other forms of assisted conception, is also currently higher than after natural fertilization, but it may decrease as techniques improve.

Multiple pregnancy (such as twins, triplets)

There is a somewhat higher risk of miscarriage in multiple pregnancies than when only one fetus is present. The likelihood of miscarriage is greater with identical twins than with non-identical twins, and also increases with the number of fetuses.

In summary, most miscarriages happen long before the fetus is capable of independent existence (Table 1). It may not be very comforting to hear that the cause is usually unknown, but fortunately in the majority of cases there is a very good chance that a subsequent pregnancy will be successful.

Table 1 Approximate frequency of miscarriage at different times in pregnancy

	Approximate % of pregnancies lost through miscarriage
Post-fertilization, pre-implantation	Not known
Post-implantation to 4 weeks' gestation[a]	10–30
4–13 weeks' gestation	10–20
14–24 weeks' gestation	2–3

[a] 4 weeks' gestation means 4 weeks after the last menstrual period, i.e. 2 weeks after fertilization. Implantation occurs approximately one week after fertilization.

• •

Having had one child already I was really confident with my second pregnancy. Unfortunately when I was eight weeks pregnant I started to bleed. My consultant arranged for me to have a scan in the Early Pregnancy Unit. By this time, I half expected something must be wrong, but thought and hoped that maybe it was my imagination. When I had the scan I was told that the fetal heart was not beating and that my cervix was open which confirmed that a miscarriage was going to occur. This was a great shock to me and I was overcome by grief at the loss of the baby.

Fortunately the medical staff were very sympathetic and they spent time with me, and reassured me that I should not blame myself for what had happened. They explained to me that the scan showed that the pregnancy had not developed as it should have and they arranged for me to have a D&C. I also had another discussion with my consultant (the author), who reassured me that there is a very good chance that my next pregnancy will be successful, which was encouraging to know, as by then I had lost my confidence in having another successful pregnancy. It was good to be able to talk to somebody who understands why miscarriages occur and I felt less guilty knowing that this could happen to anybody.

• •

At the time of writing this woman is 32 weeks pregnant in her third pregnancy which is proceeding normally.

7 *The causes of spontaneous miscarriage*

Although knowledge about the causes of miscarriages has increased considerably in recent years, there is still a great deal to be learnt. In most cases it will not be possible to be certain why a particular miscarriage occurred. Fortunately in most cases the next pregnancy will result in the birth of a live healthy baby irrespective of the cause of the miscarriage.

Causes of very early pregnancy loss

Before a period is missed

Little is known about the causes of very early pregnancy loss because it has only recently been possible to diagnose pregnancy before a menstrual period has been missed, by very sensitive measurements of hormone levels. It is likely that there are many causes of such pregnancy loss, some of which are also involved in causing miscarriages after pregnancy has been confirmed.

Causes of miscarriage in confirmed pregnancies

Doctors often divide miscarriages in confirmed pregnancies into first trimester losses (before 14 weeks' gestation) and second trimester losses (after 14 weeks' gestation). Miscarriages are much less common after 14 weeks' gestation, and it is more likely that a specific cause, other than a chromosomal abnormality, will be identified for a second trimester than for a first trimester miscarriage. There is, of course, some overlap between the causes of first and second trimester miscarriages. The more specific causes of second trimester (mid-pregnancy) miscarriages are discussed in the next chapter (Chapter 8).

Causes of first-trimester and some second-trimester miscarriages

Chromosomal abnormalities

Chromosomal abnormalities are the single most common cause of miscarriage. As described in Chapter 2, errors can occur at different stages when the chromosomal material is being rearranged. Such errors probably happen in about 1 in 10 confirmed pregnancies. In several large studies a fetal chromosomal abnormality was found in approximately half of spontaneous miscarriages for which medical advice was sought, and in which a search for a chromosomal abnormality was made. Most chromosomal abnormalities are so severe that the fetus does not survive, and the great majority of fetuses with abnormal chromosomes are miscarried spontaneously, before the end of the first trimester.

Several different types of chromosomal abnormality occur. These arise at different phases of the life of the egg, from the time that the mother was herself a fetus to the time of ovulation, and at conception when the egg fuses with the sperm. Most chromosome abnormalities arise when there is no history of genetic disease in the family, and little is known about what causes them other than that increasing age of the mother is certainly associated with an increased risk of fetal chromosomal abnormality. In some rare cases, one of the parents has a 'balanced' rearrangement of their chromosomes whereby material from one chromosome is attached to another chromosome (translocation). Fortunately, most fetal chromosomal abnormalities do not recur in the next pregnancy.

Chromosomal abnormalities in a miscarriage can sometimes be detected in a laboratory by examining cells cultured from the placental tissue. After 1–4 weeks of culture it may be possible to examine the chromosomes and to look for signs of damage. Such tests are difficult and expensive to do and are often unsuccessful. For this reason, and because most chromosome abnormalities arise spontaneously and do not recur in later pregnancies, the tests are not often performed.

Other fetal abnormalities

It is likely that many miscarriages are due to severe problems with
the development of the fetus (such as with development of the heart
or nervous system), or to serious biochemical disorders. These may
be impossible to diagnose in early pregnancy even after a miscarriage
has occurred, and the incidence of such abnormalities is therefore
unknown.

Hydatidiform mole

A hydatidiform mole is an abnormal development of the placenta. It
occurs in Britain and North America in about 1 in 2000 pregnancies,
but is much more common in the Far East. The term hydatidiform
refers to the fact that the abnormal placental (molar) tissue contains
many small grape-like fluid-filled vesicles.

The first indication that something is wrong is usually the
occurrence of vaginal bleeding. This may not start until the second
trimester of pregnancy (after 14 weeks' gestation). The diagnosis
is most frequently made by performing an ultrasound scan which
shows a 'snow-storm' appearance, and in most cases no fetus. Once
the diagnosis is certain the uterus should be emptied, usually by
suction aspiration under general anaesthesia. There is a small risk
that some abnormal placental tissue may remain and grow, occasionally developing into a rare form of cancer (choriocarcinoma)
during the following months. Fortunately, if this does happen it can
be detected by measuring human chorionic gonadotrophin (hCG)
levels in the urine or blood, and effective treatment is available.
Women are therefore asked to provide such samples for at least
a year after they have had a hydatidiform mole and to make sure
that they do not become pregnant during that time.

Increasing maternal age

Most studies have shown an increased risk of miscarriage in older
women, particularly over the age of 38 years. Miscarriages occur in
approximately 1 in 5 pregnancies at the age of 39 years, and probably
in more than half of confirmed pregnancies in women over 42 years

of age. This is partly because of the known increased incidence of fetal chromosomal abnormalities with increasing maternal age, which has led to the offer of amniocentesis or chorionic villus sampling (CVS) to women in their forties and late thirties. At the age of 38 the incidence of chromosomal abnormality at 16 weeks' gestation is about 1 in 200, and at the age of 45 it is approximately 1 in 20. It is obviously much higher earlier in pregnancy, as most chromosomally abnormal fetuses will be lost long before 16 weeks' gestation.

Other reasons for the increased risk of miscarriage in older women are less easy to evaluate. It is possible that some women conceiving late are relatively less fertile than other women, and that there is an association between their subfertility and their miscarriages.

Abnormality of the uterus

Many women with a uterine abnormality such as a congenitally abnormally shaped uterus or a fibroid uterus, do not have any problems in pregnancy but these abnormalities, and the much less common problem of intrauterine adhesions, can occasionally cause miscarriages in both the first and second trimesters of pregnancy. They are discussed more fully in the next chapter.

Intrauterine contraceptive device

The risk of miscarriage in women who have used an intrauterine contraceptive device (coil/IUCD) is not increased, provided that the device is removed before conception. If conception occurs with a device in place, there is a significant risk of intrauterine infection and of miscarriage if the strings of the device are protruding through the cervix. These risks can be reduced by gentle removal of the device by a doctor in early pregnancy.

Oral contraceptive pill

The likelihood of miscarriage is not increased in women who were taking oral contraceptive pills before they became pregnant.

Maternal diseases

Diseases affecting the mother may occasionally cause miscarriages in either the first or second trimesters.

Infections

Most maternal infections do not cause any harm to the fetus but any really severe generalized infection, such as influenza or malaria, may lead to fetal death and miscarriage.

Some infections which do not cause severe symptoms in the mother are known to cause an increased risk of fetal abnormality and of spontaneous miscarriage when they occur in early pregnancy. Steps are taken to try to reduce the likelihood of these infections arising.

Rubella (German measles) It is well known that rubella infection in early pregnancy often causes severe fetal abnormality and even fetal death followed by miscarriage. Considerable success in reducing the incidence of rubella in pregnancy has followed the widespread vaccination of children, and of women who were not already immune to rubella. However, it is very important that vaccination programmes are maintained, and that if possible a woman's immunity to rubella is checked *before* she tries to conceive so that she can be immunized at least one to two months before conception if she is found not to be already immune. Most women are checked routinely during pregnancy so that they can try to avoid coming into contact with people with rubella if they are not immune and so that can be offered immunization after delivery. Obviously, it is preferable that immunity should be checked *before* pregnancy when possible.

Syphilis Syphilis is uncommon but if this infection is present in the mother it can have devastating effects on the fetus, causing either fetal death and late abortion or a variety of congenital abnormalities. Fortunately treatment of the mother with penicillin early in pregnancy is usually effective in preventing infection of the fetus. Although syphilis is uncommon, it is tested for routinely in most pregnant women as intrauterine syphilis is so serious, if untreated, and is so easy to treat if it is diagnosed in time.

Other maternal diseases   Chronic maternal diseases rarely cause spontaneous miscarriage but there are some conditions in which the fetus is particularly at risk throughout pregnancy. These conditions include severe hypertension (raised blood pressure), severe renal (kidney) disease, diabetes and some uncommon conditions such as phenylketonuria and systemic lupus erythematosus. Women with these conditions are likely to be already under medical care. They, and women with other medical disorders such as epilepsy, should talk to the doctor who is looking after them before embarking on a pregnancy so that the possible risks can be explained to them and their treatment can be modified if necessary.

Drugs

Drugs seldom cause miscarriage, but several drugs can cause fetal abnormalities if taken during early pregnancy. It is therefore very important that women should not take any drugs that are not essential in early pregnancy. This also means that they should not take such drugs when they are trying to conceive, as the pregnancy will probably have been present for at least two weeks before they have any suspicion that they may be pregnant. As mentioned above, women who are on medical treatment should discuss their treatment with their doctor before embarking on a pregnancy.

Operations in early pregnancy

Most types of surgery in early pregnancy do not increase the risk of miscarriage, but it is sensible to postpone any non-essential surgery at least until after the first trimester or preferably until after the baby is born.

Previous operations involving the cervix

Previous termination of pregnancy is associated with a slightly increased risk of mid trimester miscarriage, due to a weakening of the cervix, known as an 'incompetent cervix' (see Chapter 8), but this problem has become less common with modern methods of termination of pregnancy.

The cervix may also rarely become incompetent following a cone biopsy operation which is occasionally performed for a woman with an abnormal smear test result to remove the area in which abnormal cells are present.

Alcohol

There is good evidence that excessive maternal alcohol intake during pregnancy increases the risk of fetal abnormality. It is likely that miscarriages are also more common in women who drink excessively. The term fetal alcohol syndrome is used to include the severe fetal abnormalities that can occur in the babies of women who drink very heavily (the equivalent of about eight glasses of wine a day). It is likely that fetal abnormalities also occur in women who drink less heavily and less frequently and it is not clear what a 'safe' level of alcohol intake is in early pregnancy. This may vary from one person to another, and clearly many women who drink the equivalent of one or two glasses of wine a day have completely normal babies. The best advice at the present time, however, must be either not to drink alcohol at all, or to drink very little both *before* conception and during pregnancy.

Smoking

It has been found that the fetuses of women who smoke are likely to grow less well than those of women who do not smoke. Some studies have also shown an increased rate of miscarriage in women who smoke heavily. It is sensible to stop smoking both *before* conception and during pregnancy.

Medical radiation

It is unlikely that any single X-ray or other diagnostic radiological investigation causes an increase in the incidence of fetal abnormality, or of miscarriage. However, in order to minimize any possible risk from exposing a developing embryo to radiation, most abdominal X-rays in women in the reproductive age group are performed only in the first 10 days of the menstrual cycle, and not at all during the first three months of pregnancy.

Visual display units

Studies done with women using visual display units (VDUs) have shown no association between the use of VDUs and pregnancy loss.

Diet

Diet before and during early pregnancy is obviously important, but it is not clear whether a poor diet is an important cause of miscarriage in the western world at the present time. In the absence of adequate knowledge on this subject it seems sensible for women hoping to become pregnant to have a well-balanced diet both before conception and during pregnancy.

It is currently recommended that women who are trying to become pregnant should take at least 400 μg folic acid a day because folic acid is essential for the normal development of the embryo. It is present in many food stuffs, particularly liver and green vegetables, and is also available in tablet form.

Immunological factors

These are discussed in Chapter 9.

Stress

It is possible that stress occasionally plays a part in causing a miscarriage to occur. This has been shown in some animal studies, but it is not so easy to evaluate in humans.

Paternal factors

These are obviously very important but they are even more difficult to assess than maternal factors. The quality of the semen can be influenced by illness and by drugs (including alcohol and nicotine) but examination of the semen is not helpful in determining the cause of miscarriages at the present time.

Environmental factors

Many studies have been performed to try to assess the influence of environmental factors (such as chemicals and radiation) on the miscarriage rate in certain at-risk populations. These studies are difficult to perform well, and have usually been based on interviews and questionnaires which rely on recall of past events, with inadequate documentation of miscarriages. It is likely that some chemicals can cause an increased rate of miscarriage in women who are exposed to them in early pregnancy. It is also possible that the wives of men who work with certain chemicals may have an increased miscarriage rate, but so far few definite associations have been found. Several studies have, however, shown a possible increased risk of miscarriage in nurses and women anaesthetists working frequently with anaesthetic gases in early pregnancy, but other studies have failed to confirm these findings. Clearly, further well-designed studies of such environmental hazards are very important.

8 *Miscarriage in mid-pregnancy*

Most miscarriages occur in the first three months of pregnancy, and a specific cause is seldom found unless a fetal chromosomal abnormality is specifically looked for. Miscarriages after the first three months of pregnancy are much less common, and when they do occur it is more likely that a specific cause will be found and that effective action may be able to be taken to reduce the likelihood of a further late (second trimester) miscarriage in a subsequent pregnancy. Some of the causes of late miscarriage are shown in Table 1. Clearly many of the other factors mentioned in the previous chapter may also cause second trimester miscarriages.

Incompetent cervix

This term is used to describe a condition in which the tissues of the cervix are unable to maintain closure of the internal os of the cervix (see Chapter 2, Figure 1) during mid-pregnancy, so that a miscarriage inevitably occurs unless measures are taken to prevent it (Figure 1). Cervical incompetence is probably responsible for approximately 1 in 10 second-trimester miscarriages. In most cases a fairly clear

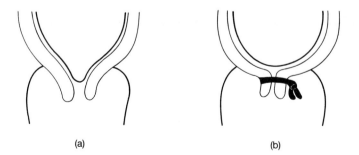

(a)   (b)

Figure 1 (a) Membranes protruding through an incompetent cervix in mid-pregnancy; (b) incompetent cervix closed by cervical suture.

Table 1 Some causes of late (second trimester) miscarriage

Structural abnormality of reproductive tract
  Cervical abnormality – incompetent cervix
  Uterine abnormality – congenital abnormality
                       uterine fibroids
                       intrauterine adhesions

Rupture of the membranes and infection

Multiple pregnancy

Factors leading to fetal death in the second trimester
  Chromosomal or other congenital abnormality
  Placental separation
  Rhesus disease
  Maternal illness

Following diagnostic tests
  Amniocentesis
  Fetoscopy
  Chorionic villus sampling (CVS)
  Cordocentesis

sequence of events precedes the miscarriage and the diagnosis can be made with reasonable certainty. In other instances, however, the diagnosis may not be so clear cut.

Cervical incompetence is not usually congenital, which means it is not usually a condition that is present from birth. Most often it is caused by instrumental dilatation of the cervix, or less frequently by other operations on the cervix such as a cone biopsy in which a cone-shaped piece of the cervix is removed. It is seldom caused by a routine 'dilatation and curettage' (D and C), or hysteroscopy, as the cervix is not usually dilated very much during these procedures. Most frequently it is caused by forceful over stretching of the internal os of the cervix. Some years ago some gynaecologists thought that severe dysmenorrhoea (painful periods) in adolescents could be relieved by forceful dilatation of the cervix with disruption of the cervical tissue around the internal os. It has been realized, however, that not only is this operation ineffective treatment for dysmenorrhoea, but that it can actually damage the cervix and render it incompetent, and so the operation is no longer performed. Nowadays the commonest surgical cause of an incompetent cervix is a vaginal termination of pregnancy, during the course of which the cervix is dilated more than during a routine D and C, to allow removal of the fetus and placenta. The later the pregnancy is terminated, the more the cervix has to be dilated. Gynaecologists are well aware of the possibility of damaging the cervix during termination of pregnancy operations and take care to avoid causing such damage. The tissues of the cervix can also occasionally be damaged during a difficult delivery of a baby, but significant damage to the cervix during delivery is uncommon.

The typical sequence of events that occurs during pregnancy when the cervix is incompetent is as follows. The pregnancy usually proceeds normally until some time during the second trimester when, most commonly between the sixteenth and twenty-fourth weeks of pregnancy, there may be an increase in the normal vaginal mucous discharge, and a feeling of heaviness in the vagina for a few days as the cervix shortens and begins to dilate. Then, often with very little warning and with few contractions, the cervix opens further and the pregnancy is expelled. The membranes may rupture first, allowing amniotic fluid to escape, or the sac may be expelled intact with the baby inside it. The placenta may or may not be expelled. The baby will be the appropriate size for the length of gestation and will usually be alive and completely normal, but too immature to survive. If the placenta is not expelled soon after the baby it may be necessary to remove it under anaesthesia. The picture may be much less clear than this and it may be difficult to know whether or not a miscarriage was due to an incompetent cervix. It is very important to decide whether this was the cause; if it was, late miscarriages will continue to occur in all subsequent pregnancies unless appropriate action is taken to support the cervix. Fortunately effective treatment is available, but this will not prevent miscarriages due to other causes, and it should only be used when it is likely that the cervix is incompetent.

Treatment of incompetent cervix

The aim of treatment is to support the internal os, and to prevent it dilating until towards the end of the third trimester. Several operations have been devised to achieve this aim. The ones most commonly performed consist of the insertion of a non-absorbable tape round the cervix at the level of the internal os (Figure 1). This operation is often called 'insertion of Shirodkar (or McDonald) stitch, or suture' after two of the doctors who described such an operation. The stitch is usually put in at about the fourteenth week of pregnancy after the danger of a first trimester miscarriage (which is never due to an incompetent cervix) has passed and before the danger of a miscarriage due to an incompetent cervix arises.

The woman is admitted to hospital for the operation, which is usually performed through the vagina, under a general anaesthetic. She may be kept in hospital for a few days afterwards. She is then able to go home and to resume her normal activities. She will usually be advised to refrain from sexual intercourse for about two weeks or occasionally longer. The operation is simple and seldom causes any serious problems. Often there will be increased vaginal discharge during the pregnancy because of the presence of the suture material, but usually no other side effects occur. The stitch is normally very effective if the right diagnosis was made. Occasionally, however, a miscarriage or preterm labour may occur despite the insertion of a stitch, and it is vitally important that the woman should return to hospital if she has any vaginal bleeding, leakage of fluid, or uterine contractions. If miscarriage or preterm labour is occurring the stitch will have to be removed.

Ideally the stitch should remain in place until about the thirty-eighth week of pregnancy. It is then removed as it is no longer required and the chances of normal labour starting increase day by day. Removal is simple and does not usually require an anaesthetic. A speculum is inserted into the vagina; the stitch can be seen, and is easily held with forceps and cut with scissors and removed. The woman is then able to go home to await the normal onset of labour. A stitch will be required in all subsequent pregnancies.

Unfortunately the diagnosis of incompetent cervix is usually only made after a second trimester miscarriage has occurred, with loss of the baby. Very occasionally the diagnosis is made in pregnancy before a miscarriage occurs, if the cervix is found to be dilating. It is sometimes possible to save such a pregnancy by inserting a stitch after the cervix has already begun to dilate. There are no reliable tests that can be performed between pregnancies to make a certain diagnosis of incompetent cervix.

If the cervix is very damaged it may be necessary to insert the stitch using the abdominal route. If this is done the baby will be delivered by caesarean section.

Abnormalities of the uterus

Abnormalities of the shape of the cavity of the uterus may be congenital (present from birth) or due to the presence of fibroids in the wall of the uterus or much less commonly to adhesions in the uterine cavity.

Congenital abnormalities of the uterus

These are fairly common; they are probably present in about 1 in 100 women. Many different abnormalities can occur. They usually arise because of the way in which the uterus develops in a female fetus, being formed by fusion of two hollow ducts. The walls of the ducts normally break down where they are in contact with one another to form the uterus, so that there is normally only one uterine cavity with a fallopian tube on each side. Failure of development of one duct, or of fusion of the ducts, or failure of breakdown of the adjoining walls after fusion, can occur, leading to a variety of uterine abnormalities, some of which are depicted in Figure 2.

Congenital uterine abnormalities, particularly a T shaped uterus, have also been found to occur in some of the daughters of women who were treated with diethylstilboestrol (DES) in pregnancy. DES is a synthetic oestrogen which was given to pregnant women, mainly in the United States in the 1950s, for a variety of conditions associated with pregnancy. Problems in the daughters of these women came to light in the 1970s; doctors have been advised not to prescribe DES in pregnancy for many years.

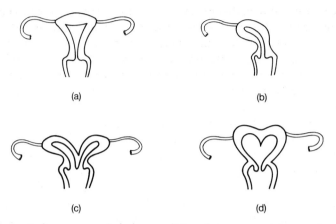

Figure 2 Some congenital abnormalities of the uterus: (a) normal uterus; (b) unicornuate (one-horned) uterus; (c) bicornuate (two-horned) uterus; (d) uterus with septum.

The diagnosis of a congenital uterine abnormality is sometimes made on vaginal examination—if for example a double vagina or double cervix is present—but these particular abnormalities are uncommon, and the diagnosis is more often made on ultrasound examination or by undertaking an X-ray examination known as a hysterosalpingogram, or by performing a hysteroscopy.

A hysterosalpingogram is an X-ray examination which is designed to give information about the cavity of the uterus and the state of the fallopian tubes. It is usually performed in an X-ray department, without an anaesthetic. It is important that it is performed in the follicular phase of the menstrual cycle, that is soon after the end of a period and before ovulation, so that there is no risk of irradiating a fertilized ovum or embryo. Following a vaginal examination, a speculum is introduced into the vagina, and the cervix is grasped gently to steady it. This may cause some discomfort. A small tube is then introduced into the cervical canal so that dye which will show up on an X-ray can be injected into the cavity of the uterus and along the fallopian tubes. At the same time as the dye is injected the abdomen is screened, using an X-ray machine, and the dye can be seen on a nearby television screen filling and outlining the cavity of the uterus and then flowing along the tubes. Two or three X-ray pictures are usually taken so that there is a permanent record of the findings (Plate 3). The instruments are then removed and the woman is able to go home after a short rest. Discomfort similar to a period pain is commonly experienced as the dye enters the uterus; it is usually short lived. A pain killer can be taken to relieve the discomfort, if necessary.

A diagnostic hysteroscopy is a procedure in which a very fine telescope (hysteroscope) is passed through the cervical canal and into the uterine cavity. This can usually be done as an outpatient procedure, without an anaesthetic. The walls of the uterus can be thoroughly checked and the openings of the fallopian tubes into the uterus can be seen. Congenital abnormalities of the uterus, polyps, and submucous fibroids and intrauterine adhesions can be diagnosed. Some of these can be dealt with using an operating hysteroscope. A general anaesthetic is often given when an operating hysteroscope is used.

In many cases uterine abnormalities cause no problems during pregnancy, but problems can occasionally arise. Rarely, a uterine abnormality such as a bicornuate uterus will cause recurrent miscarriages but more often a miscarriage in someone with a uterine abnormality is due to a cause other than the abnormality. In most cases the pregnancy will proceed normally. I have even delivered normal healthy twins from a woman with a completely bicornuate (two horned) uterus—there was a baby in each uterine horn!

In a very few women who have recurrent miscarriages a uterine abnormality is the cause, and occasionally it may be appropriate to have an operation to correct the abnormality. Sometimes the operation can be performed using an operating hysteroscope but it may be necessary to perform an abdominal operation and to cut into and therefore to scar the uterus and this can cause problems, including infertility and in a subsequent pregnancy. Such operations are not often undertaken.

Fibroids

Fibroids are very common non-malignant tumours that arise in the muscular wall of the uterus. They are rare before the age of 20 years but become increasingly common as women grow older, and are present in at least 1 in 5 women by the age of 40 years. They can vary in number from one to more than a hundred, and in size from less than the size of a pea to more than the size of a melon. Most often, however, they are less than 10 in number and smaller than a grapefruit.

No one knows why they arise or how to prevent them occurring. They are slightly more common in women who have not been pregnant than in those who have, and they are known to occur more commonly in women of African descent than in Caucasian women. However, they are found frequently in women of all races whether or not they have been pregnant. They may be in the wall of the uterus (intramural) or they may protrude into either the uterine cavity (submucous fibroids and fibroid polyps) or more commonly into the abdominal cavity (subserous fibroids) (Figure 3). They may cause considerable enlargement of the body and cavity of the uterus. Subserous and intramural fibroids are usually diagnosed by abdominal or vaginal examination. Submucous fibroids and fibroid polyps can be diagnosed by hysterosalpingography or hysteroscopy. Most fibroids can be seen on ultrasound examination.

Many women with fibroids become pregnant and have no problems from the fibroids. Occasionally, however, fibroids may

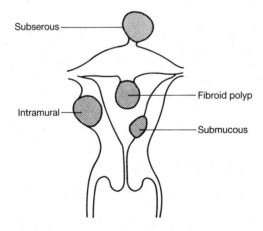

Figure 3 Some possible sites for uterine fibroids.

cause a problem early in pregnancy or later on. Possible early pregnancy problems that may arise with a fibroid polyp or submucous fibroid include failure of implantation and early or late miscarriage. Problems that can arise later on in pregnancy are outside the scope of this book. It is unusual for fibroids to be the cause of recurrent miscarriages, and it is likely, if a woman with fibroids has one or even two miscarriages, that they are caused by something other than the fibroids. However, if a woman is found to have a fibroid polyp it should certainly be removed, whereas removal of a submucous fibroid may or may not be advisable depending on whether it has caused problems or not. Fibroid polyps can usually be removed vaginally; the method of removal will depend on their size and whether or not they have caused the cervix to dilate. If the cervix has dilated they can often be removed during a D and C; if the cervix has not dilated, they will usually be removed using an operating hysteroscope. Submucous fibroids can also often be removed nowadays using an operating hysteroscope.

In summary, fibroids are common but they seldom cause miscarriages unless they protrude into the uterine cavity. If they do protrude into the uterine cavity removal of the fibroids may be advisable.

Intrauterine adhesions

These are uncommon. They can occur following curettage of the uterus, particularly when it is performed within three or four weeks of the end of a pregnancy. If a woman who has miscarried or who is infertile is found to have intrauterine adhesions, it may be possible to break them down using an operating hysteroscope, but unfortunately treatment is not always successful, and the woman may remain infertile or she may have further miscarriages.

Rupture of the membranes and infection

The membranes can rupture ('the waters' can break) at any time during the second and third trimesters of pregnancy, leading to either a gush of amniotic fluid or to a lesser but persistent loss of fluid. In many cases the reason why the membranes rupture is not clear but it has been shown that infection can sometimes weaken the membranes and cause them to rupture.

If the waters break the woman should be admitted to hospital and swabs should be taken from the cervix to determine whether infection is present. The woman should rest, mainly in bed, and she should be monitored for signs of infection by having her temperature and pulse rate checked, noting any symptoms of abdominal discomfort and the nature of the fluid lost, and by gentle abdominal palpation.

In some cases the membranes will seal over again without any evidence of infection and the pregnancy will proceed normally; in other cases labour will ensue or infection will become apparent. If labour starts following rupture of the membranes there is little chance of stopping it and delivery of the baby is likely to occur. If the pregnancy is less advanced than 24 weeks it is very unlikely that the baby will survive, but if it is 24 weeks or more, a paediatrician should be present at the delivery to allow the baby to have the best possible chance. If intrauterine infection becomes established it will be necessary to induce labour because of the great danger of maternal septicaemia (blood poisoning) which may follow intrauterine infection. Antibiotics are unlikely to save the life of a fetus that becomes infected in the uterus following rupture of the membranes, and they may also be ineffective in controlling maternal infection if the woman remains undelivered. If there are signs of intrauterine infection, in the presence of ruptured membranes in a woman who is less than 24 weeks pregnant, an intravenous syntocinon drip will usually be commenced to stimulate labour.

The earlier in pregnancy that the membranes rupture the less likely is the pregnancy to continue successfully. I have, however, looked after one woman whose membranes ruptured at 16 weeks' gestation and who leaked fluid continuously for the next 14 weeks; her membranes then sealed over and she eventually delivered a healthy baby at term.

Multiple pregnancy

The risk of miscarriage in mid-pregnancy increases with an increasing number of fetuses. The risk is also higher in a twin pregnancy

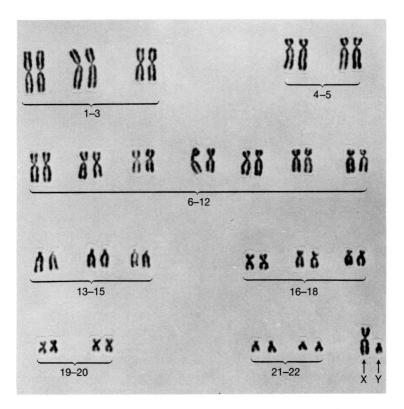

PLATE I. The 23 pairs of chromosomes of a normal male.

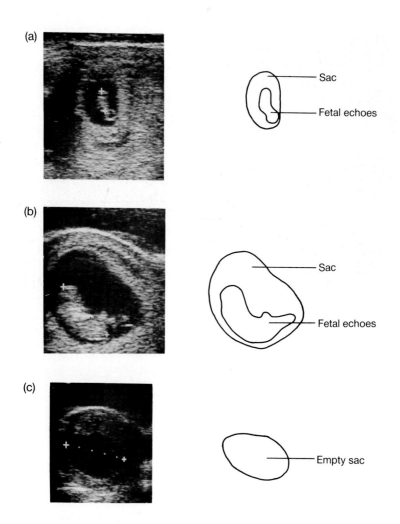

PLATE 2. (a) Ultrasound scan at 7 weeks' gestation showing normal fetal echoes. (b) Ultrasound scan at 10 weeks' gestation showing normal fetal echoes. (c) Ultrasound scan showing empty sac. The crosses on the scans are the markers that are used for making measurements.

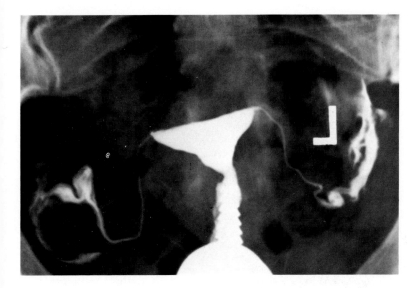

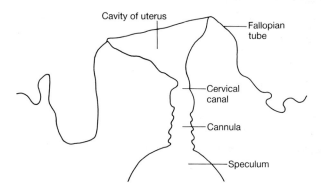

Cavity of uterus

Fallopian tube

Cervical canal

Cannula

Speculum

PLATE 3 (*a*). Normal hysterosalpingogram. A speculum is inserted into the vagina and dye that will show up on an X-ray is run via a cannula (metal tube) into the cervical canal and thence into the cavity of the uterus and along the Fallopian tubes.

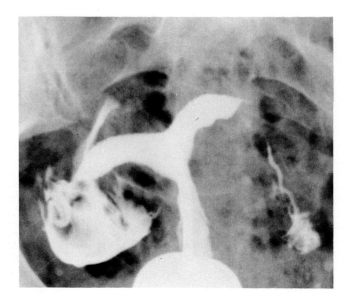

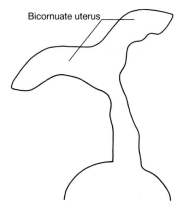

Bicornuate uterus

PLATE 3 (*b*). Hysterosalpingogram showing bicornuate uterus.

when the fetuses are identical (formed from one fertilized egg) than when they are not identical (formed from two fertilized eggs).

Factors leading to death of the fetus in the second trimester

Chromosomal or other congenital abnormality

Most severe chromosomal and other fetal abnormalities lead to miscarriage in the first trimester, but occasionally they will cause death of the fetus and miscarriage in the second trimester.

Separation of the placenta

First-trimester miscarriages usually start with vaginal bleeding and abdominal pain, caused by separation of some or all of the placenta from the wall of the uterus, before the pregnancy is expelled. Separation of the placenta before expulsion of the fetus is much less common in the second and third trimesters, but it may occur, and it is then usually referred to as placental abruption. There may only be a small area of placental separation and the pregnancy may continue normally. On the other hand, there may be sufficient separation of the placenta to cause fetal death, or to cause the uterus to contract and the cervix to dilate, with delivery of the baby.

If bleeding occurs during the second trimester of pregnancy a doctor should be contacted. If the baby is alive the woman should rest in bed, and other causes of vaginal bleeding should be excluded. There is a good chance that the bleeding will settle and that the pregnancy will continue normally. If it is thought that some placental separation has occurred, the pregnancy should be monitored more closely than usual to make sure that placental function remains normal.

Rhesus incompatibility

This is an uncommon cause of fetal loss in the second trimester and has become even less common since the widespread administration of anti-D to women at risk of developing anti Rhesus positive (anti-D) antibodies. Rhesus incompatibility arises when a Rhesus-positive fetus is carried by a Rhesus-negative mother who has developed anti-Rhesus positive antibodies. These antibodies can cross the placenta and cause breakdown of fetal red blood cells, thus causing fetal anaemia and sometimes fetal death in either the second or, more often, the third trimester. The antibodies usually develop in response to the leakage of some Rhesus- positive fetal red cells into the mother's circulation at the time of a previous delivery or miscarriage or at the time of amniocentesis or chorionic villus sampling (see Chapter 11). It has been found that the administration of anti-D to Rhesus-negative women at risk, at the time of each delivery or miscarriage, and during pregnancy, greatly reduces the likelihood of the production of anti-Rhesus positive antibodies by the mother, and so Rhesus incompatibility is becoming much less common.

If a baby is lost in the second trimester because of Rhesus incompatibility, the baby will have died before the miscarriage occurs. The woman should be very carefully monitored during the next pregnancy by checking amniotic fluid samples taken by amniocentesis (see p. 80). If it is found that she is once again carrying a severely Rhesus-affected baby, intrauterine transfusion with Rhesus negative red cells may be indicated. A special needle containing a very fine plastic tube is passed, under local anaesthetic, through the mother's abdominal wall and through the wall of the uterus into the baby's umbilical cord, or abdominal cavity, using ultrasound to visualize the baby. The needle is withdrawn and Rhesus-negative red cells are then slowly transfused into the baby through the fine plastic tube. Other blood group incompatibilities may also cause recurrent fetal problems and can be managed in a similar way.

Illness in the mother

Some of the illnesses in the mother which may harm a fetus are discussed in Chapter 7.

Miscarriage following diagnostic tests

Amniocentesis, fetoscopy, chorionic villus sampling (CVS), and cordocentesis

These tests are described in Chapter 11. The risk of miscarriage due to amniocentesis is approximately 1 in 200, and that due to fetoscopy is approximately 1 in 30. The newer technique of chorionic villus sampling (CVS) which is performed earlier in pregnancy at about 10 weeks' gestation, has reduced the need for the later tests to be performed in women at increased risk of fetal abnormality. The chance of miscarriage following CVS is thought to be about 1 in 50 to 1 in 30. The risk of fetal loss following cordocentesis is approximately 1 in 100 to 1 in 50.

Photographs of the baby

Many parents find it helpful to have a photograph of their baby if it dies in the uterus and is stillborn, or if it dies following delivery (neonatal death) in the third trimester. The photographs can help the parents to grieve. The same can be true for a couple who have lost a baby in the second trimester and they may want to create a book of memories which might include an early ultrasound picture, photographs of the baby, and cards and letters sent by relatives and friends.

• •

I knew quite a few friends who had experienced problems conceiving and so I was amazed to find that at the age of 38 I had no such difficulty. However, six weeks later I had my first miscarriage. Subsequently a number of people told me of their miscarriage experiences. This I found quite surprising as nobody had ever spoken to me about them before. It was as if they were something that should remain hidden and only spoken about in whispers. After the first miscarriage 18 months passed before I conceived again, although I often felt pregnant. I lost this pregnancy at seven weeks as I did another, three months later. I began to wonder if I would ever have a baby. Had my age beaten me or had the fibroids, which had been discovered, caused my system to fail? I had become very tense about the whole situation with life being ruled by the monthly cycle.

One of the aspects I found most hurtful was the attitude of other people. Seemingly intelligent people would make such tactless comments as, 'When are you going to start a family?', 'Any news yet?', 'You'd make good parents'. I started to adopt various tactics in order to avoid any possible reference to babies in conversation.

Throughout the experience the doctors have been supportive. Not discounting me but being matter of fact, and trying to ascertain what may have been the problem, and in dealing with each complication sympathetically.

By the time I conceived for the fourth time we viewed the whole process very sceptically. Each day was counted off, each sign of pregnancy noted while constantly looking for indications that the pregnancy might fail again. We couldn't believe it when I successfully completed 12 weeks. I found it difficult to look positively on the pregnancy but as each week passed we became more hopeful.

Unfortunately I went into labour early, at 27 weeks, but I gave birth to a perfect baby girl who needed very little help and who has progressed remarkably well. In the end it has all been worth while but the experience has given us a different perspective on the whole business of having children.

• •

9 *Recurrent miscarriages*

• •

Recurrent miscarriages can cause immeasurable unhappiness and despair to the couples who are unfortunate enough to experience them. All the emotions that may be engendered by a single miscarriage (as discussed in Chapter 5) are likely to be even more intense, and it becomes very difficult for the couple to believe that they will ever have a healthy baby. Fortunately, however, even after three consecutive miscarriages the next confirmed pregnancy has a better than 1 in 2 (50%) chance of ending with the birth of a live healthy baby, without any treatment. Even after four, five, or more miscarriages the chance of a successful pregnancy is still greater than 4 out of 10 (40%).

The underlying cause of each successive miscarriage is not necessarily the same. As chromosomal and other fetal abnormalities are so common in early pregnancy, it is possible for a woman to have a fetus with a chromosomal abnormality in one pregnancy and then a different problem in her next pregnancy, by chance. For these reasons, and because it is usually not possible to find a treatable cause of miscarriage, most couples who have had less than three consecutive miscarriages are not offered tests or treatment. The exception is if there appears to be a clear-cut reason for the miscarriages, such as an incompetent cervix, or there is some reason to believe that the woman has a medical disorder which could cause recurrent miscarriages. Even after three consecutive miscarriages it is unlikely that any specific abnormality will be detected and, as mentioned above, the chance of a successful pregnancy is still good. However, in some couples who have three consecutive miscarriages a significant abnormality will be found, and it is therefore sensible to consider investigation after three consecutive miscarriages. If a problem is found it may be possible to correct it. If no problem is identified the couple will usually feel reassured and more able to contemplate a further pregnancy.

Possible causes of recurrent miscarriages

Some factors which may cause recurrent miscarriages are given in Table 1, but there is still uncertainty about the importance of some of these factors.

Genetic factors

Parental chromosomal rearrangement

As discussed in Chapter 7, it has been found that the fetal chromosomes are abnormal in at least half of clinically recognizable first trimester miscarriages. Usually the next pregnancy will be chromosomally normal, but in a very few cases the abnormality is due to a parental chromosomal rearrangement and a further fetal chromosomal abnormality may occur. The risk of this happening when one parent has a chromosomal rearrangement is variable. The likelihood of finding a parental chromosomal abnormality in a couple who have had three consecutive miscarriages is less than 1 in 20, but it is appropriate for all couples who have had three miscarriages to have their chromosomes checked. Blood samples are taken into special tubes from both parents and are taken to a specialized laboratory for chromosome analysis.

The couple should see a genetic counsellor for advice if one of them is found to have a chromosomal abnormality. In most cases there is a reasonable chance that a normal baby will be conceived. The fetal chromosomes can be checked in pregnancy, if the parents wish this to be done, either by CVS or amniocentesis (see Chapter 11).

Table 1 Some possible causes of recurrent miscarriages

Genetic factors	Immunological factors
Cervical or uterine abnormality	Rhesus incompatibility
Hormonal deficiency	Infection
Maternal medical disorder	

Other genetic factors

If the parents' chromosomes are normal, there is still a chance of the baby being affected by other genetic disorders such as neural tube defects. These include spina bifida and anencephaly, which arise when the spinal cord and brain do not develop properly. If a couple have had one fetus with a neural tube defect, they have a risk of approximately 1 in 20 of conceiving another fetus with a neural tube defect. Neural tube defects in a fetus can usually be detected on an ultrasound scan performed at 19 weeks' gestation.

If it is found that recurrent miscarriages are due to a genetic problem on the father's side artificial insemination of donor semen (AID) may be considered. Ovum donation is a possibility if a genetic problem is found on the mother's side but it is a much more complex and expensive undertaking than AID, and the success rate is of the order of only 1 in 5 for each attempt.

Cervical and uterine abnormalities

These are discussed in Chapter 8. The diagnosis of cervical incompetence is usually easily made from a knowledge of the history of the miscarriages: they usually occur after 14 weeks' gestation and are relatively rapid and pain free. There is usually a loss of mucus but no bleeding beforehand, and the baby is normal and the appropriate size for the dates. Treatment is with a cervical suture in the next pregnancy.

Abnormalities of the uterus are a fairly uncommon cause of recurrent miscarriage, but after three miscarriages an ultrasound examination and a hysterosalpingogram or hysteroscopy (see p. 54) may be performed, so that the shape and cavity of the uterus can be visualized. Abnormalities that may be detected include a congenitally abnormally shaped uterine cavity, submucous fibroids or fibroid polyps and, rarely, adhesions inside the uterus. If a fibroid polyp is found it should be removed; this can usually be done using an operating hysteroscope. Other abnormalities must be carefully evaluated before deciding whether treatment is advisable or not. Most women with either fibroids or a congenitally abnormally shaped uterus do not have an increased likelihood of miscarriage and do not require any treatment.

Hormonal deficiency

Progesterone is a hormone produced by the ovary and later by the placenta. It plays an important role in preparing the endometrium for implantation and in maintaining pregnancy. It is possible that there may sometimes be inadequate progesterone production in early pregnancy and that this could lead to early miscarriages, which could be recurrent. It is difficult to prove that this is the case, but several studies have shown somewhat low levels of progesterone after ovulation, and/or inadequate development of the endometrium, in a few women with recurrent miscarriages.

Progesterone levels can be increased either by treatment with a drug called clomiphene, during the early part of each menstrual cycle (which will cause the ovary to produce more progesterone after ovulation) or with progesterone pessaries or suppositories, in the second half of the cycle and in early pregnancy. Successful pregnancies have followed both these forms of treatment. However, as mentioned earlier, even after three consecutive miscarriages there is at least a 50 % chance of a successful pregnancy without treatment, and so it is hard to be sure whether the good outcomes were due to the treatment or not. There have been no adequate trials of these forms of medication, and the possible risks of medication must be weighed up against the possible benefits in each particular case.

There is some evidence that an increased level of luteinizing hormone (LH) in the first half (follicular phase) of the cycle may be associated with an increased chance of miscarriage. High follicular phase levels of luteinizing hormone are commonly found in women with polycystic ovaries and these women are known to have an increased risk of miscarriage. Research is continuing in this area.

Maternal medical disorders

These are usually apparent in their own right and are discussed in Chapter 7.

Immunological factors

The science of immunology has developed very rapidly in recent years and is continuing to do so. It is known that all human beings possess a very large number of cellular antigens (substances which provoke antibody formation) from an early stage of development. These antigens can stimulate an antibody response in other human beings if tissue is transplanted from one person to another, as in a kidney or heart transplant, and are responsible for the tissue rejection that may occur after such transplant operations.

Antigens are also very important in pregnancy. In a normal pregnancy the fetus will possess antigens from the father as well as the mother, and it might therefore be expected that the fetus would be rejected by the mother's body, just as transplanted tissue is rejected if the recipient's immune system is not suppressed with drugs. The reason that not all fetuses are rejected is that immunological changes occur in a normal pregnancy that prevent the mother's body from rejecting the fetus. It has been thought by some people that too many identical antigens should not be present in both the mother and the father, because when they are these immunological changes may not be stimulated, and recurrent miscarriages may then occur. Some women suspected of having such an immunological problem as the cause of recurrent miscarriages have had successful pregnancies following treatment with transfusions of white blood cells. However, as discussed before, the success of these pregnancies may not have been due to the treatment. Controlled studies are being performed to assess the value of this form of therapy in couples who have had several miscarriages, and in those who are found to share several antigens, and to make sure that the treatment has no disadvantages. The place of this form of treatment has yet to be established.

Anticardiolipin antibodies

Occasionally recurrent miscarriages can be due to the presence of a substance known as an antiphospholipid or anticardiolipin antibody or lupus anticoagulant, in the mother's blood. This should be tested for after two or three early or later pregnancy losses in which intrauterine death has occurred. Treatment may involve low dose aspirin therapy or sometimes treatment with corticosteroids or low dose heparin.

Rhesus incompatibility

This is discussed in Chapter 8. Severe Rhesus and other blood group incompatibilities can very occasionally cause recurrent miscarriages in the second trimester of pregnancy.

Infection

General infections

Although a general infection such as rubella (German measles) may cause a miscarriage if the mother develops it during early pregnancy, there is no definite evidence that infections other than untreated syphilis can cause recurrent miscarriages.

Local infections

As discussed in Chapter 8 rupture of the membranes in the second trimester can be associated with local cervical infection. It is therefore important for this to be considered in a woman who has had a second trimester miscarriage following rupture of the membranes, and for cervical swabs to be taken if appropriate.

Possible investigations in a couple who have had recurrent miscarriages

It is very important that a full and clear history of all the mother's pregnancies and of her present and past health is obtained and that she is examined thoroughly before deciding which, if any, further investigations are appropriate. A detailed family history should also be obtained from both members of the couple, as this may reveal a genetic factor.

Investigations that may be recommended include chromosome analysis of both parents, blood grouping and testing for blood group antibodies and for anticardiolipin antibodies, hormone estimations, ultrasound examination of the reproductive organs, and hysterosalpingography or hysteroscopy (Table 2).

Chromosome analyses require special laboratory facilities but

Table 2 Possible investigations in a couple who have had recurrent miscarriages

---

In all cases
    full medical, gynaecological, and obstetric history
    family history
    general and vaginal examination, with cervical swabs if indicated

In appropriate cases
    chromosome analysis of both parents
    blood group and blood group antibodies
    anticardiolipin antibodies
    hormone estimations
    ultrasound examination
    hysterosalpingogram/hysteroscopy

---

they do not cause much inconvenience to the couple, as all that is required is a straightforward blood sample. This is also the case for checking the blood group and testing for blood group antibodies, and for detecting anticardiolipin antibodies. Hormonal evaluation may entail measurement of luteinizing hormone levels in the first half of the menstrual cycle and of progesterone levels in the second half of the cycle and in early pregnancy, and possibly the measurement of other hormone levels as well. Most hormone estimations are carried out on blood samples. At the present time detailed immunological evaluation is only undertaken in a few centres. The techniques of hysterosalpingography and hysteroscopy have been described earlier (p. 54).

Treatment possibilities in couples with recurrent miscarriages

As mentioned at the beginning of the chapter, a couple who have had three consecutive miscarriages for no obvious reason have at least a 50 % chance of a successful pregnancy without any treatment. This makes it very difficult to evaluate the efficacy of any particular therapy. It is very natural for couples to seek treatment and for doctors to wish to try to help with any treatment that might be of value, but this does not mean that giving treatment is necessarily the best course of action as most forms of treatment have some disadvantages.

General advice

Women who have experienced recurrent miscarriages are naturally very anxious and are usually keen to do anything that may help a pregnancy to succeed. It is obviously advisable for them to have a well-balanced diet and to avoid alcohol, smoking, and drugs at the time of conception and during early pregnancy in order to provide the best environment for the developing fetus. It is generally accepted that taking folic acid supplements daily, both before and directly after conception, reduces the risk of the fetus developing spina bifida or other neural tube defects, and there is no evidence that this does any harm. It has been given routinely, combined with iron, to reduce the chance of women becoming anaemic in pregnancy for many years, and it is routinely given in a higher dose to women with twins.

Bed rest

Women who have had recurrent miscarriages for no known reason are usually advised to rest as much as possible during early pregnancy. A few women will find it reassuring to be admitted to hospital for rest, but most will prefer to stay at home. There is no definite evidence that rest increases the successful pregnancy rate, but it is quite possible that anything that helps to reduce anxiety may occasionally be beneficial.

Sexual intercourse

The uterus contracts during orgasm and it is possible that this might increase the likelihood of miscarriage if the pregnancy is unstable. Many couples with recurrent miscarriages refrain from intercourse during early pregnancy in the hope that this will increase the chances of the pregnancy continuing. There is no definite evidence that this is in fact so, and it is probably equally important to avoid a strain on the couple's relationship. However, if bleeding has occurred it is probably wise to avoid intercourse for at least two weeks afterwards, as this may be a sign that the pregnancy is already in jeopardy.

Specific treatment

If a specific cause for the recurrent miscarriages is found then the appropriate treatment should be given as described above.

Case history

The following case history may offer encouragement to women who have had several miscarriages and who find it hard to believe that they will ever have a baby.

• •

A woman of 38, whom I was looking after, had had six pregnancies in seven years and they had all ended in miscarriage—at 12, 6, 10, 6, 8 and 12 weeks' gestation respectively. No cause had been found for her recurrent miscarriages. She had had a normal hysterosalpingogram, and her chromosomes and her husband's chromosomes were normal. She was admitted to hospital at 6 weeks' gestation in her seventh pregnancy for bed rest as she was naturally very anxious. Two days later she started to have slight vaginal bleeding. This continued intermittently during the next six weeks and was sometimes associated with lower abdominal pain and the passage of small clots. At 8 weeks' gestation an ultrasound scan showed that the fetus was alive and the right size for the dates. A further scan at 12 weeks' gestation showed that the fetus was alive and growing satisfactorily. She went home at 14 weeks' gestation. Her pregnancy was straightforward from then on, and she delivered a normal healthy baby boy weighing 7 lb at 38 weeks' gestation.

She became pregnant again nine months later and was so busy with her baby that she was unable to take much extra rest during the pregnancy. She once again had some bleeding during the early weeks, but otherwise the pregnancy was straightforward. She delivered another normal healthy boy weighing 6 lb 8 oz at 38 weeks' gestation. No treatment other than rest was given in either pregnancy.

• •

10 *Pregnancy after miscarriage*
•••

The majority of women who have one, two, or even three or more miscarriages will also have successful pregnancies. You may find this hard to believe, especially after several miscarriages, but it is true.

For most women the chance of having a successful pregnancy after a pregnancy that has ended in miscarriage is very good. After one or two miscarriages, the probability of the next confirmed pregnancy ending with the birth of a live healthy baby is almost the same as if there had never been a miscarriage. After three consecutive miscarriages, the chance of the next confirmed pregnancy being successful is still greater than 1 in 2 (50 %) and even after more than three miscarriages the chance of a successful pregnancy is still greater than 4 out of 10 (40 %).

When to try again

The best time to start trying for another baby will vary from one couple to another. It is generally advisable to wait about three months to get over the physical, and more particularly, the emotional effects of miscarriage. Some couples will need more time than this to mourn the loss of the baby; if they start a new pregnancy before they have had time to work through their grief, they may experience a prolonged resumption of grief during the next pregnancy and after the birth of their new baby, and they may find it difficult to relate to the new baby.

Special precautions before conception

It is obviously sensible to try to create the best possible environment for the developing fetus. If the woman is not already immune to rubella (German measles), it is advisable for immunization to be performed soon after the miscarriage, so that two months can elapse before she tries to become pregnant again. Adequate contraceptive precautions should be taken for one to two months after rubella immunization.

The woman should have a well-balanced diet, and smoking and alcohol intake should be stopped or reduced to a minimum. No drugs that are not essential should be taken. If the woman has a medical disorder, she should discuss the management of this with her doctor before conception occurs, so that adjustments to her treatment can be made if necessary. Unnecessary stress should be avoided. It is natural for the woman to be very anxious, but her anxiety can be reduced by support and understanding from those closest to her, and sympathetic reassurance from her doctor. It is important that she should have confidence in her medical attendants. In most cases the cause of the previous miscarriage will not be known or, even if it is known, no specific treatment will be available or required. Even so, the above precautions may help to increase the likelihood of a successful pregnancy.

There is increasing evidence that taking a small amount of folic acid daily, both before and after conception, reduces the likelihood of the baby developing spina bifida (see page 47).

Advice during early pregnancy

It may be wise not to tell too many people about the pregnancy too soon in case another miscarriage does occur, even though this is statistically unlikely. It can be more upsetting for the couple if too many people know about it. On the other hand, telling close friends about the pregnancy will bring understanding and support from them, whatever the outcome.

Some women feel superstitious about admitting that they are pregnant in case this brings bad luck. Others will feel that the pregnancy is unreal anyhow, and will not be able to believe that they can carry a pregnancy successfully. They may not make any preparations for the care of the baby until late in pregnancy, or even until after the birth of the baby. It is a good idea, however, for them to make preparations, at least during the third trimester, as otherwise they may feel that the baby is unreal when it is born, and they may find it difficult to relate to the baby and to believe that it will survive.

A woman who has had a miscarriage in a previous pregnancy is likely to be very anxious, to be very easily upset emotionally, and to think a lot about her previous miscarriage. She may have nightmares about having another miscarriage. Such anxieties and strong feelings are normal, and her partner and friends should be aware of this and give her plenty of sympathy, encouragement, and support.

Sexual intercourse

It is very unlikely that sexual intercourse will harm the pregnancy, but some couples will prefer to refrain from intercourse in early pregnancy when there has been a previous early miscarriage.

Bleeding in early pregnancy

It is important to remember that many women experience bleeding in early pregnancy and do not miscarry. Once a fetal heart beat has been detected the chance of the pregnancy being successful is greater than 9 out of 10 (90 %), even when there has been some bleeding.

Specific treatment

Only very rarely does any specific treatment improve the outlook for the pregnancy. One instance where treatment is essential is if the woman has an incompetent cervix. In this instance mid-pregnancy miscarriage will inevitably occur if she does not have a cervical suture inserted (see p. 49).

In the majority of cases there is no specific treatment that will reduce the likelihood of a miscarriage occurring, but the chances of a successful pregnancy are usually good, even after three miscarriages, without any specific treatment.

● ●

I remember when I became pregnant for the first time four years ago, the mixed feelings I had about becoming a mother with all the implications that that would have had. I had just started a postgraduate course in a different country (I am from Brazil) with a prospect of considerable stress ahead. I actually did not have much time to get used to the idea of having a baby as after only a few weeks I had a miscarriage. In a way I felt relieved and I came to the conclusion that it was for the best.

Just over a year later, I became pregnant again and this time I felt more positive, thinking that although the circumstances were not ideal, we (my husband and I) wanted to do our best for the baby. We had time to think it over and the idea of having a baby seemed more and more appealing, and right for us. Everything went fine until the eleventh week, when I started bleeding in the afternoon and miscarried early the next day. It was probably the worst night I ever had, not only for the physical pain, but particularly for the feeling that it was out of our hands and there was nothing we could do. I felt very, very frustrated.

We went to the hospital in the morning and I had to have a D&C. I had to face very traumatic days afterwards, feeling without energy and not wanting to accept the fact that I had lost the baby. I thought that I was undergoing all the suffering and perhaps attributed the blame to myself. However, my husband called my attention to the fact that he also suffered and felt the same way as I did. His support was the only thing that helped me at that time. It took him quite a long time to recover, though, and for some time he felt he did not want to try again, as a measure of self protection. However, time is indeed a helpful remedy. We both felt more confident after a few months and decided we would like to try again until we felt I would be too old for it (I was 36 then). If we were not successful we would try to adopt a baby.

More recently I became pregnant for the third time, and again miscarried after only a few weeks. The process was familiar to me, but the emotional strain was overwhelming, for each time I had so much hope that everything would be all right and once again it went wrong. To put my mind at rest we went through medical examinations and tests to detect any possible cause, but nothing wrong was observed. A few months ago when we least expected it, I became pregnant again and I am very hopeful that this time I will have a successful pregnancy. I feel a lot more prepared now and I am very certain the chance of participating in the process of helping to originate life is worth taking.

• •

Scans at 8 and 13 weeks showed the baby was growing normally. The couple were very reassured by this. The membranes ruptured at 36 weeks and a healthy baby was born. Her husband was very surprised as he flew in from Brazil that day not knowing his wife was in labour! They were both delighted with their daughter.

11 *Antenatal care in early pregnancy*

For most women, no major complications occur in the first few months of pregnancy. Nonetheless, serious problems can arise and it is very important that every woman should be seen early on, or preferably before she becomes pregnant if she has any medical problems, by the doctors and midwives who are going to look after her during her pregnancy. In Britain, most women have their babies in hospital and the care of pregnant women is usually shared by the woman's general practitioner (GP), or another GP if her own GP does not undertake antenatal care, community midwives, and the doctors and midwives at the hospital where the baby is going to be born. In the United States, too, most babies are born in hospital; prenatal care may be undertaken by a private doctor, or by a team of doctors at the hospital.

In Britain, a woman should see her own GP first and discuss the arrangements for her care during pregnancy with him or her. If the pregnancy has not already been confirmed, it may be helpful to take an early morning urine specimen in a clean jar to the doctor's surgery at that time (the equivalent of half a cupful of urine is enough). The doctor can then arrange for a pregnancy test to be performed on the sample. Sometimes the test can be done immediately; sometimes the sample has to be sent away to be tested.

Your first hospital visit

Ideally you should be seen at the hospital for your first (booking) visit between 8 and 12 weeks after your last period, if you have not had any problems in this or any other pregnancy. If you have had problems it may be advisable for you to be seen sooner.

The purpose of the booking visit is literally to book a bed for the delivery and the postnatal period, as each hospital can only accommodate a certain number of patients, to check that you are healthy and that the pregnancy is proceeding normally, and to arrange for various blood tests and other investigations to be performed. Routines vary from one hospital to another, but in general you will be asked a lot of questions about your previous pregnancies, your past medical history and your family history, and you will then be asked about the present pregnancy. In some hospitals an ultrasound scan is performed at the first visit to ensure that the pregnancy is proceeding normally and to confirm the dates.

Your urine will be tested for protein and sugar and for evidence of infection. Routine blood tests will be arranged. The purpose of these is to establish your blood group and to see whether you have any abnormal antibodies (such as Rhesus antibodies which could affect the baby), to make sure that you are not anaemic, and to determine whether you are immune to rubella (German measles), as a rubella infection in early pregnancy can have very serious consequences for the fetus. A blood test to exclude syphilis is also performed routinely in most hospitals, as this infection is so dangerous for the fetus (and the mother), and so easy to treat if it is diagnosed in time. Tests for hepatitis and for the human immunodeficiency virus (HIV test) are usually also offered.

In many hospitals arrangements are made for screening tests for fetal spina bifida and Down's syndrome to be performed on a maternal blood sample taken at about 15–16 weeks' gestation. These tests are discussed more fully later in this chapter.

At the first visit, or one arranged for a few days later, you will usually be examined by a doctor. You will have a general physical examination including measurement of your weight and blood pressure, checking for any signs of ill health, and examination of your breasts and abdomen.

A vaginal (internal) examination may also be performed. Some women are unhappy about having a vaginal examination, but it can give important information that will help in the safe care of the pregnancy, and there is no evidence at all that it can harm the baby. It is important for this examination that your bladder is empty. You will be asked to lie on your back (or occasionally on your side) with your knees drawn up, as for a cervical smear test. The doctor will usually first insert a smooth metal instrument (a speculum) into the vagina in order to look at the cervix (neck of the womb). A cervical smear may be taken at this time if one has not been done recently. If there are signs of infection or if you have noticed excessive discharge, itching, or soreness, or if a previous miscarriage was thought to be possibly due to local infection, swabs may be taken for culture. The doctor will then perform an internal examination with two fingers of one hand inserted into the vagina and with the other hand on the lower abdomen, so that the uterus can be gently felt between the fingers of the two hands. The purpose of this examination is firstly to confirm that the uterus is enlarged to the expected size, and secondly to check that there is no abnormality in the reproductive organs such as uterine fibroids, an ovarian cyst, or an ectopic pregnancy (a pregnancy in one of the fallopian tubes). A preliminary assessment of the size of the birth canal can also be made at this time.

Ultrasound

If there is a difference between the size of the uterus on examination and the size that the uterus is expected to be from the date of the last menstrual period, an ultrasound scan will usually be arranged if one has not been performed already (Plate 2). In some hospitals this is now performed routinely but not all hospitals offer routine scans to all antenatal patients, although there are some advantages in doing so. For example, one of the most important things that a doctor needs to know about a pregnant woman is how far advanced the pregnancy is. This is essential if blood tests that need to be timed (such as screening tests for spina bifida and Down Syndrome, which are usually done at 15–18 weeks' gestation) are to be performed. A knowledge of the length of gestation is very important if any problems arise later in pregnancy or if the pregnancy becomes 'overdue'. It is easy to establish the duration of pregnancy fairly accurately in early pregnancy, but it becomes more difficult as pregnancy advances because different babies grow at different rates.

Transvaginal scans are being performed increasingly often in the first trimester. An ultrasound probe is inserted into the vagina, instead of moving it over the abdomen. The advantages of transvaginal scans, as opposed to transabdominal scans, are that the ultrasound pictures are better and the woman's bladder does not need to be full.

An ultrasound scan performed after 7 weeks' gestation will confirm whether the fetus is alive, as by this stage the heart can usually be seen to be beating, which is obviously very reassuring to someone who has previously had a miscarriage. Once the fetal heart beat can be seen, the likelihood of a miscarriage falls to less than 1 in 20. Should a miscarriage occur later, it will help the woman and her doctor to understand more about the type of miscarriage that she had. Follow-up scans may be performed at intervals of two to four weeks, in someone who has had more than one miscarriage, and will show whether or not the fetus is continuing to grow normally.

Screening tests for spina bifida and Down Syndrome

In some hospitals all pregnant women are offered the opportunity of having the level of alpha fetoprotein (AFP) in their blood measured as a screening test for fetal spina bifida and other neural tube (spinal cord and brain) defects. In other hospitals the test is only offered to women who have already had a fetus with a neural tube defect or who have a family history of such a problem. If the fetus has a neural tube defect the level of AFP in the mother's blood will usually be higher than normal between 15 and 18 weeks' gestation. This test is not intended to give a diagnosis of neural tube defects, but to detect women at risk. Other things can affect the result. For example, the mother's dates may be wrong, there may be a fault in the laboratory measurement, or the level may be raised for a reason other than a fetal neural tube defect (such as a twin pregnancy or bleeding earlier in pregnancy), or for no obvious reason. If the level is found to be raised, a repeat measurement may be arranged and an ultrasound scan will be performed to check the dates, to exclude twins, and to look at the fetus with particular reference to the spine and the head, to make sure that they are developing normally. A few women will then be offered an amniocentesis (see below) so that the AFP level in the amniotic fluid can be measured, as this will give a more accurate prediction of a fetal problem than measurement of the AFP level in the mother's blood.

It has been found that there is an association between low levels of AFP in maternal blood and Down Syndrome, and also between high levels of human chorionic gonadotrophin (hCG) and Down's syndrome (known as the Double Test). If levels of both AFP and hCG are measured in maternal blood samples, taken between 15 and 18 weeks' gestation, the combined result will be found to be abnormal in about two-thirds of pregnancies in which the fetus has Down Syndrome. In the Triple test oestriol levels are also measured.

When the doctor or midwife discusses with you whether you would like to have your blood AFP and hCG levels measured, they should make it clear to you that if abnormal levels are found, this does not necessarily mean that there is anything wrong. Otherwise you will understandably be even more anxious than necessary if someone telephones you and asks you to come for a discussion. Most hospitals contact women when the likelihood of spina bifida or Down Syndrome is more than 1 in 200. Only in a small number of women who are recalled will there actually be a serious problem with the fetus.

Amniocentesis

Amniocentesis is the name given to the test that is performed when a sample of the amniotic fluid around the baby is taken for analysis, usually at about 15–16 weeks' gestation. The test does carry a risk of miscarriage (about 1 in 200). It is therefore only offered to women at increased risk for chromosome disorders such as Down Syndrome, and other abnormalities. A pool of fluid is located using an ultrasound scanner and amniotic fluid is then withdrawn via a fine needle, inserted through the mother's abdominal wall. It used to be normal practice to use a local anaesthetic before inserting the needle but many obstetricians no longer do this, as the discomfort of inserting the local anaesthetic is often as great as the insertion of the amniocentesis needle. Culture of the cells in amniotic fluid takes up to three weeks and in about 1 in 50 cases a result cannot be obtained.

Later in pregnancy amniocentesis can be used to determine the severity of Rhesus disease in a woman with Rhesus antibodies (see p. 59). The risk from an amniocentesis later in pregnancy is less than with an amniocentesis at 16 weeks.

Fetoscopy

In this investigation, a thin lighted telescope is introduced into the amniotic sac through the mother's abdominal wall under local anaesthesia, at about 18 weeks' gestation, in order to look at either the fetus or the fetal blood vessels. A sample of fetal blood or even fetal tissue can be obtained for analysis in order to detect certain fetal abnormalities in cases at risk. This investigation carries a greater risk of causing miscarriage than amniocentesis (about 1 in 30) and is therefore only used in exceptional circumstances.

Chorionic villus sampling (CVS)

This is a newer technique in which a small sample of chorionic villi (the microscopic finger like processes that form the main substance of the placenta) is obtained after 10 weeks' gestation under sterile conditions. The sample may be taken via the cervical canal (transvaginal CVS) or via the mother's abdominal wall (transabdominal CVS). The advantage of CVS is that a result is obtained earlier in pregnancy than with amniocentesis but it carries a higher risk of miscarriage than amniocentesis (about 1 in 30 compared to 1 in 200).

Cordocentesis

In this technique a sample of the baby's blood is obtained from the umbilical cord via the mother's abdominal wall, under ultrasound control. It is rarely undertaken, but when necessary it can be performed in the second or third trimester. It carries a risk of fetal loss of about 1 in 100 to 1 in 50.

Some do's and don'ts in early pregnancy

Diet and drugs

It is advisable to have a well-balanced diet, to stop smoking, and to reduce alcohol consumption before conception occurs. No unnecessary drugs should be taken by someone who is trying to conceive. If drugs are needed for the treatment of a medical disorder, it is very important for these to be discussed with your GP or with the hospital doctor who is looking after you, so that any necessary changes can be made, before conception. As discussed earlier it is advisable to make sure that an adequate amount of folic acid is taken daily both before conception and during early pregnancy (see page 47).

Exercise

There is no evidence that moderate exercise does any harm in early pregnancy and you can safely continue your usual forms of activity unless these are very strenuous or dangerous, or any complications of pregnancy arise. Thus there is no reason why you should not continue with such activities as walking and swimming. Undue exhaustion should, however, be avoided.

Sexual intercourse

This is very unlikely to cause any harm to the pregnancy unless there has been any bleeding. It may, however, be best for someone who has had several early miscarriages to abstain from intercourse in early pregnancy.

Announcing the pregnancy

You may prefer not to tell too many people too soon about the pregnancy in case a miscarriage does occur—it can make it even more distressing if too many people know about the pregnancy. On the other hand, support from close friends is very important if a miscarriage does occur, and therefore there is no reason why they should not know about the pregnancy from an early stage.

Most women who have had one or more early miscarriages will wait until after 13 weeks' gestation or more, and until they have had a normal ultrasound scan, before they tell many people about the pregnancy. Under these circumstances the chances are very good (more than 95 %) that you will have a live healthy baby.

Useful addresses

Other parents who have suffered a loss have formed associations to help those in similar situations. The following associations produce helpful information and can put you in touch with their members. Sometimes it may be helpful for a nurse, doctor, or counsellor to make the initial contact for you. Do not hesitate to ask you would like them to ring up for you.

United Kingdom

Miscarriage Association
c/o Clayton Hospital
Northgate, Wakefield
West Yorkshire
WF1 3JS
Tel: 01924 200 799

Sands
Stillbirth and Neonatal Death
Society
28 Portland Place
London W1N 4DE
Tel: 0171 436 5881

Satfa
Support around Termination for
Abnormality
73 Charlotte Street
London W1P 1LB
Tel: 0171 631 0285

Tamba – Bereavement Group
Twins and Multiple Births
Association
PO Box 30
Little Sutton
South Wirral
L66 1TH
Tel:0151 3480020

USA

MIDS Inc. (Miscarriage, Infant
Death, Stillbirth)
c/o Janet Tischler
16 Crescent Drive
Parsippany, NJ 07054
Tel: 201 966 6437

Pregnancy and Infant Loss Center
1421 East Wayzata Boulevard
Wayzata, MN 55391
Tel: 612 473 9372

Pregnancy Loss Support Program
National Council of Jewish
Women, NY Section
9 East 69th Street
New York, NY 10021
Tel: 212 535 5900

Share
Pregnancy and Infant Loss
Support, Inc.
St Joseph Health Center
300 First Capitol Drive
St Charles, MO 63301
Tel: 314 947 6164

DES Action USA
Long Island Jewish Hospital
New Hyde Park, NY 11040
Tel: 516 775 3450

Glossary

• •

Technical words have usually been defined in the text where they first occur. They can be traced by using the index. Some of them are also defined here for easy reference.

Abortion (miscarriage): The loss of a pregnancy from the uterus before 20–24 weeks' gestation (see Chapter 1).

Alpha fetoprotein (AFP): Fetal protein normally found in very small amounts in the mother's blood. The mother's blood level of AFP may be measured at about 15–16 weeks' gestation; it is usually raised when the fetus has spina bifida, and with a twin pregnancy; it is often decreased when the fetus has Down Syndrome (see p. 79).

Amniocentesis: A procedure in which a fine needle is passed through the mother's abdominal wall into the amniotic sac in order to obtain a sample of amniotic fluid for analysis (see p. 80).

Amniotic fluid: The fluid surrounding the fetus.

Amniotic sac: The sac, formed by the amnion and chorion (membranes), in which the fetus lies inside the uterus.

Antibodies: Substances produced by the body to protect it against infection and some other foreign substances (antigens).

Anti-D: Anti-Rhesus positive (D) antibodies that can destroy Rhesus-positive red blood cells (see p. 59).

Antigen: A substance which provokes antibody formation by the body.

Blighted ovum: A pregnancy in which the fetus ceases to develop very early on. The amniotic sac may only contain fluid and no fetal tissue when the miscarriage occurs. This term is seldom used nowadays; a better term is early embryonic loss or demise.

Blood groups: The main blood groups which are tested for in pregnancy are the ABO and Rhesus blood groups. Everyone has either A, B, O, or AB blood and is either Rhesus-positive or Rhesus-negative.

Cervical canal: The passage through the cervix connecting the body of the uterus and the vagina (see Figure 1 in Chapter 2).

Cervix: The neck of the womb (uterus) (see Figure 1 in Chapter 2).

Chorionic villus: (singular); **chorionic villi** (plural): Microscopic finger-like processes which form the main substance of the placenta (afterbirth).

Chromosomes: Structures, each consisting of two connected rods which are made up of thousands of genes, which transmit all the hereditary information necessary for the development and formation of the tissues of the body. Every human cell (other than the ova and sperms) normally contains 23 pairs of chromosomes (see Plate 1).

Complete abortion/miscarriage: All the products of conception are expelled from the uterus and a curettage is not necessary.

Cone biopsy: An operation in which a cone-shaped piece of cervical tissue is removed. It is sometimes performed when a cervical smear shows abnormal cells.

Congenital: Present at birth.

Cordocentesis: This is a technique in which fetal blood is taken from the umbilical cord, through the mother's abdominal wall, under ultrasound control (see p. 81).

Corpus luteum: 'Yellow body'. A structure formed in the ovary from an ovarian follicle from which ovulation has occurred.

Dilatation and curettage (D and C): A minor operation in which tissue is removed from the inside of the uterus (a scrape).

Ectopic pregnancy: A pregnancy growing outside the uterus, usually in one of the fallopian tubes (see p. 16).

Embryo: The developing baby in early pregnancy.

Endometrium: The lining of the uterus.

Fallopian tubes: The tubes that form a passage from the ovaries to the uterus (see Figure 1 in Chapter 2)

Fertilization: The fusion of an ovum (egg) and a sperm.

Fetoscopy: A specialized test in which a fine lighted telescope is inserted into the amniotic sac so that the fetus, or the fetal blood vessels in the umbilical cord or on the surface of the placenta can be visualized (see p. 81).

Fetus: The baby while still in the uterus.

Fibroids: Common non-malignant tumours that arise in the muscular wall of the uterus.

Follicle: An ovarian follicle consists of an ovum (egg) and the layers of cells that surround it.

Follicle-stimulating hormone (FSH): A hormone secreted by the pituitary gland, which initiates the development of one or more ovarian follicles.

Follicular phase: The part of the menstrual cycle which precedes ovulation.

Genes: The minute units of which the chromosomes are made up. They carry all the hereditary information necessary for the development and function of the tissues of the body.

Genetic counsellor: A doctor who is qualified to discuss with couples who are, or who may be, at extra risk of having a child with an inherited disorder what the risk is and what the consequences might be, and whether there are any tests that could be done in pregnancy to show whether the fetus has the disorder.

Hormone: A chemical messenger that is made in one part of the body and affects the functions of cells in various parts of the body.

Human chorionic gonadotrophin (hCG): A hormone produced by the placenta. Detection of this hormone forms the basis of the standard pregnancy test.

Hydatidiform mole: An abnormal development of the placenta (see p. 42).

Hysteroscopy: An operation in which a fine telescope is passed through the cervical canal into the uterus in order to visualize the uterine cavity. It can be performed with or without an anaesthetic (see p. 55).

Hysterosalpingogram: An X-ray examination in which the inside of the uterus and the fallopian tubes can be visualized (see p. 54).

Incomplete abortion/miscarriage: Only some of the products of conception have been expelled and some tissue remains in the uterus.

Induced abortion: An abortion that is caused intentionally.

Intrauterine transfusion: A procedure in which compatible blood is given to the fetus, usually via a very fine plastic tube inserted through the mother's abdominal wall and the uterus directly into a fetal blood vessel or into the fetal abdominal cavity (see p. 60).

Laparoscopy: An operation in which a lighted telescope is introduced into the abdominal cavity so that the uterus, ovaries and tubes can be seen (see p. 17).

Luteinizing hormone (LH): A hormone secreted by the pituitary gland. The increased release of this hormone on about day 12 to 13 of a normal menstrual cycle causes ovulation to occur approximately 24 hours later.

Membranes: The two layers of tissue forming the wall of the amniotic sac. The inner one is called the amnion and the outer one the chorion.

Miscarriage (abortion): The loss of a pregnancy from the uterus before 20 to 24 weeks' gestation.

Missed abortion: The fetus has died but a miscarriage has not yet occurred.

Mucus: A sticky substance produced by certain tissues, such as the glands in the cervical canal.

Myomectomy: An operation in which fibroids are removed (and the uterus is not removed).

Neural tube: The tissue from which the spinal cord and brain develop in the embryo (see **Spina bifida**).

Oestrogens: One of the two types of female hormones produced by the ovary and placenta. The other female hormone is progesterone.

Ovum (singular); **ova** (plural): An egg (female reproductive cell).

Pituitary gland: A small (about 1 cm diameter) but very important structure lying in the middle of the skull under the lower surface of the brain. It exerts control over several other glands by the production of hormones (see p. 5).

Placenta (afterbirth): The structure attaching the umbilical cord and the fetus to the wall of the uterus, through which the fetus obtains its nutrients and oxygen and through which its excretory products are transferred to the mother. The placenta also makes several hormones.

Pregnancy test: A test for pregnancy based on the detection of human chorionic gonadotrophin in the urine.

Products of conception: The fetus, placenta, and amniotic sac.

Progesterone: A hormone which is produced in increasing quantities by the ovary after ovulation and by the placenta during pregnancy.

Progestogen: Progesterone and progesterone-like drugs.

Rhesus antibodies: Antibodies produced by a Rhesus-negative person in response to the presence of Rhesus-positive red blood cells in his/her body (see p. 59).

Rubella: German measles. A viral disease which may cause severe fetal abnormalities if contracted in early pregnancy.

Salpingitis: Inflammation of the fallopian tubes.

Septic abortion/miscarriage: An abortion/miscarriage accompanied by infection of the cavity of the uterus.

Speculum: An instrument which, when inserted into the vagina, allows the vaginal walls and cervix to be seen.

Sperm: A male reproductive cell.

Spina bifida: A condition in which some of the bony elements of the spine fail to join, leaving part of the spinal cord and its coverings exposed.

Suction aspiration: A method of emptying the uterus via the cervical canal.

Threatened abortion/miscarriage: The occurrence of vaginal bleeding during the first 20–24 weeks of pregnancy.

Trimester: Pregnancy is divided into three trimesters or terms. The first ends at 14 weeks' gestation, the second ends at 28 weeks' gestation, and the third ends with delivery.

Ultrasound: High frequency sound waves which can be used to visualize the uterus, the placenta, the amniotic fluid, the fetus, and many other structures.

Uterus: Womb (see p. 4).

Weeks of pregnancy/gestation: The number of weeks since the first day of the woman's last menstrual period, assuming that she has an approximately 28-day menstrual cycle.

Womb: Uterus (see p. 4).

Index

••